Systemic Corticosteroids for Inflammatory Disorders in Pediatrics

Rolando Cimaz
Editor

Systemic Corticosteroids for Inflammatory Disorders in Pediatrics

Adis

Editor
Rolando Cimaz
AOU Meyer
Pediatric Rheumatology
Firenze
Italy

ISBN 978-3-319-16055-9 ISBN 978-3-319-16056-6 (eBook)
DOI 10.1007/978-3-319-16056-6

Library of Congress Control Number: 2015941518

Springer Cham Heidelberg New York Dordrecht London

Printed on acid-free paper

Adis is a brand of Springer
Springer International Publishing AG Switzerland is part of Springer Science+Business Media (www.springer.com)

Contents

1935, he began collaborating with E.C. Kendall to identify this substance. Kendall isolated four adrenal cortical hormones by 1935, which he named compounds A, B, E, and F. Subsequently, it was demonstrated that Kendall's compound E and Hench's substance X were the same. Eight years later they extracted small quantities of compound E (named cortisone by Hench) for clinical trials. T. Reichstein perfected techniques for manufacturing adrenal hormones, heralding a new era in therapeutic pharmacology [4].

The first patient treated with cortisone (1948) was affected by rheumatoid arthritis; soon thereafter other patients with rheumatic diseases received cortisone or adenocorticotropic hormone. Oral and intra-articular administration of cortisone and hydrocortisone began in 1950–1951, while the semisynthetic production of cortisone started in 1952. Pediatric experience with corticosteroids also started in these years: for example, in 1951 the *British Medical Journal* described five children (three with rheumatoid arthritis, one with acute rheumatic carditis, one with nephrosis) treated with oral cortisone [5]. In the same year, seven other children with nephrotic syndrome were treated with cortisone [6]. Between 1954 and 1958, six synthetic steroids were introduced for systemic anti-inflammatory therapy. Corticosteroids were rapidly adopted as a beneficial treatment in patients with rheumatic diseases, as well as in patients with asthma and allergies, soon after the first report of their good effects in patients with rheumatoid arthritis in 1949 [7]. However, by 1960 all of the toxic effects of long-term corticosteroid administration and the protocols to withdraw such drugs while minimizing symptoms of cortical insufficiency had been described. Thereafter, the discovery of new drugs (such as nonsteroidal anti-inflammatory drugs and methotrexate) progressively reduced the role of steroid therapy in rheumatic diseases [2].

Even from the first report on the effects of cortisone in patients with rheumatoid arthritis, it was obvious that side effects were going to be a limiting factor in the use of this drug for long periods of time [1]. Table 1 summarizes the historically reported side effects associated with steroid therapy [8]. Since the 1950s, clinicians searched for new therapeutic strategies to limit the systemic side effects of corticosteroids, such as the administration of corticosteroid joint injections in patients with rheumatoid arthritis [9]. However, even if intra-articular steroid administration is generally considered as a safe procedure, sometimes it can be contraindicated or cause side effects (Table 2) [10]. Regarding oral steroid therapy, an alternate-day regimen was developed to reduce the systemic effects. The alternate-day regimen was demonstrated to be effective in maintaining suppression of disease activity but not in preventing its exacerbation. Moreover, the alternate-day regimen could not be used to induce suppression or to treat exacerbations. Whenever a patient on alternate-day therapy relapses, daily steroid therapy should be resumed until the disease is controlled [8]. To reduce the systemic effects of steroid treatment, topical steroid therapy was developed. For example, inhaled corticosteroids have been particularly favored because they provide a targeted anti-inflammatory benefit to the airways without subjecting patients to major systemic effects. However, even inhaled corticosteroids are not completely void of systemic or local side effects at higher doses in some patients.

Table 1 Historically reported side effects of systemic steroid therapy [8]

Inhibition of growth
Osteopenia–osteoporosis (impaired peak bone mass accrual in childhood and adolescence)
Hypertension
Fluid retention
Hypokalemic alkalosis
Weight gain
Hyperlipidemia
Diabetes mellitus
Avascular necrosis of bone
Nephrocalcinosis
Uricosuria
Poor wound healing
Ecchymosis
Skin atrophy and striae rubra
Pseudotumor cerebri
Psychosis, euphoria, depression
Pancreatitis
Hepatomegaly
Increased susceptibility to infections
Reactivation or dissemination of viral or fungal infections
Posterior subcapsular cataract
Glaucoma
Hematologic changes (erythrocytosis, thrombocytosis, leukocytosis)
Proximal myopathy
Steroid withdrawal syndrome (fever, anorexia, nausea, lethargy, arthralgia, desquamation of the skin, weakness, and weight loss)

Table 2 Intra-articular steroid injections: contraindications and side effects [10]

Contraindications
Unstable joints–Charcot neuroarthropathy
Local infection: periarticular sepsis (especially when there is high risk of causing spread to joint)
Local infection: septic arthritis
Bacteremia
Intra-articular fracture (acute)
Failure to respond to prior injections
Blood clotting disorders
Side effects (*rare*):
Septic arthritis
Postinjection flare
Atrophic changes
Systemic absorption (suppression of hypothalamic–pituitary axis)
Soft tissue calcinosis

Among the reported side effects of corticosteroids, growth retardation is of particular concern and specific for pediatric age. A small yet clinically significant and persistent growth retardation is possible with long-term use of inhaled corticosteroids in childhood, even at low-to-medium doses. Nevertheless, these findings should be weighed carefully against the potential for greater growth retardation that might result should frequent asthma exacerbations occur by withholding inhaled corticosteroid therapy, thus necessitating frequent oral corticosteroid bursts [11]. Indeed, the evidence for oral corticosteroids and their effects on growth is unambiguous [12–15].

Besides growth retardation, long-term use of corticosteroids in childhood and adolescence may impair the physiological process of bone mass accrual and the attainment of peak bone mass, leading to an increased risk of osteoporosis later in life. Existing data suggest that the relationship between inhaled corticosteroid use and bone mineral density in children is conflicting and confounded by numerous other variables and awaits further evaluation. On the contrary, chronic and even intermittent use of oral corticosteroids has the potential to cause a decrease in bone mineral density and increase the risk for osteoporosis and fractures in both children and adults. Therefore, clinicians should carefully weigh the potential benefit against this risk before prescribing long-term or short-term oral corticosteroid therapy [11].

Steroid administration has been proposed for several pediatric diseases, with conflicting results. In 1975, more than 25 years after their discovery, Walton and Ney wrote, "When administered for other than adrenocortical replacement, corticosteroids are not ideal therapeutic agents because at best one may hope for suppression of a disease process but rarely, if ever, a cure." Authors have also reported that corticosteroids are relatively benign when given in large doses for a few days but are associated with severe toxic effects when administered continuously [16]. Interestingly, in 1985 Spirer and Hauser reported again that "except for the few indications for replacement steroid therapy, the rest are still controversial. Even when the use of corticosteroids in a certain disorder is widely accepted, the preferred regimen may still be debatable. Uncontrolled anecdotal data have seeded much confusion about the real indications for steroid therapy, and created fear of its effects." They also reported that "whenever steroid therapy may be avoided or replaced by less harmful non-steroidal drugs, the latter is preferable. A local steroid preparation is preferable to systemic therapy (such as inhaled corticosteroids for asthma or intranasal steroids for allergic rhinitis). Moreover, whenever possible a 'steroid-saving' policy should be used by the addition of non-steroidal preparations. Indeed, in any case the benefit from therapy should outweigh the side effects, and the preparation with the best therapeutic index should be used" [8]. Table 3 presents the diseases for which corticosteroids were proposed until 1985. Despite this large number of conditions, only in a few was the evidence in favor of administering steroids sufficient to universally recommend steroid treatment. Nowadays many studies are still conducted to evaluate the efficacy of corticosteroids in the treatment of several diseases, a large number specific for pediatric age. Table 4 lists reviews published in the Cochrane Library in the period 2013–2014, confirming that the debate and the interest regarding the therapeutic role of corticosteroids is still a matter of concern [17–34]. The indication for steroid administration changed

Table 3 Diseases for which steroid treatment was proposed until 1985 [8]

Neuromuscular disorders
Guillain–Barré syndrome
Bell's palsy
Myasthenia gravis
Duchenne muscular dystrophy
Sydenham's chorea
Opsoclonus
Infantile spasms (West syndrome)
Pseudotumor cerebri
Hypernatremic dehydration
Acute bacterial meningitis
Acute meningoencephalitis
Brain tumors
Respiratory disorders
Asthma
Bronchiolitis
Allergic bronchopulmonary aspergillosis
Sarcoidosis
Cardiovascular disorders
Acute viral myocarditis and pericarditis
Rheumatic carditis
Hematologic and oncologic disorders
Idiopathic (immune) thrombocytopenic purpura
Autoimmune hemolytic anemia
Diamond–Blackfan syndrome
Paroxysmal nocturnal hemoglobinuria
Immune neutropenia
Pediatric oncology
Renal disease
Nephrotic syndrome
Renal transplant rejection
Gastrointestinal disorders
Acute fulminant liver failure
Chronic active hepatitis
Inflammatory bowel disease
Collagen and rheumatic diseases
Systemic lupus erythematous
Polyarteritis nodosa
Mixed connective disease
Kawasaki disease
Stevens–Johnson syndrome
Schönlein–Henoch purpura
Allergic disorders
Allergic rhinitis
Acute anaphylaxis
Acute urticaria
Chronic urticaria or angioedema

(continued)

Table 3 (continued)

Dermatologic disorders
Capillary-cavernous hemangiomas
Toxic epidermal necrolysis
Alopecia areata
Contact dermatitis
Atopic and seborrheic dermatitis
Psoriasis
Ophthalmologic diseases
Bacterial conjunctivitis
Viral conjunctivitis
Chronic herpetic keratitis
Allergic conjunctivitis
Episcleritis
Uveitis
Optic neuritis
Infections
Pertussis
Typhoid fever
Infectious mononucleosis
Septic shock
Replacement therapy
Congenital adrenal hyperplasia
Adrenal insufficiency
Other indications
Neonatal hypoglycemia
Malignant hyperthermia

Table 4 Reviews on steroid treatment published in the Cochrane Library, 2013–2014

Disease	Study	Year of publication	Reference
Acute bacterial meningitis	Corticosteroids for acute bacterial meningitis	2013	[17]
Acute sinusitis	Intranasal steroids for acute sinusitis	2013	[18]
Acute viral bronchiolitis	Glucocorticoids for acute viral bronchiolitis in infants and young children	2013	[19]
Asthma	Ciclesonide versus other inhaled corticosteroids for chronic asthma in children	2013	[20]
Asthma	Combination formoterol and budesonide as maintenance and reliever therapy versus current best practice (including inhaled steroid maintenance) for chronic asthma in adults and children	2013	[21]
Asthma	Combination formoterol and budesonide as maintenance and reliever therapy versus combination inhaler maintenance for chronic asthma in adults and children	2013	[22]

Table 4 (continued)

Disease	Study	Year of publication	Reference
Asthma	Intermittent versus daily inhaled corticosteroids for persistent asthma in children and adults	2013	[23]
Bronchiectasis	Combination inhaled corticosteroids and long-acting β2-agonists for children and adults with bronchiectasis	2014	[24]
Chronic lung disease in preterm infants	Early (<8 days) postnatal corticosteroids for preventing chronic lung disease in preterm infants	2014	[25]
Chronic lung disease in preterm infants	Late (>7 days) postnatal corticosteroids for chronic lung disease in preterm infants	2014	[26]
Cough (subacute cough)	Inhaled corticosteroids for subacute cough in children	2013	[27]
Crohn's disease	Budesonide for maintenance of remission in Crohn's disease	2014	[28]
Cystic fibrosis	Oral steroids for long-term use in cystic fibrosis	2013	[29]
Cystic fibrosis	Topical nasal steroids for treating nasal polyposis in people with cystic fibrosis	2013	[30]
Postoperative ear discharge	Interventions for the prevention of postoperative ear discharge after insertion of ventilation tubes (grommets) in children	2013	[31]
Preterm birth	Different corticosteroids and regimens for accelerating fetal lung maturation for women at risk of preterm birth	2013	[32]
Preterm birth	Thyrotropin-releasing hormone added to corticosteroids for women at risk of preterm birth for preventing neonatal respiratory disease	2013	[33]
Viral myocarditis	Corticosteroids for viral myocarditis	2013	[34]

also for diseases in which it seemed revolutionary, because of the development of new drugs with more efficacy and fewer side effects. Before the introduction of corticosteroids, children with arthritis faced a lifetime of pain and disability. Whereas corticosteroids were once the mainstay of therapy, today they are largely used as bridge or adjunctive therapies [35, 36]. However, with time, corticosteroids have acquired an important role in other diseases. For example, the 2014 UK guidelines for Kawasaki disease suggested the addition of corticosteroids to intravenous immunoglobulin in severe cases with the highest risk of intravenous immunoglobulin resistance [37]. Finally, corticosteroids have been proposed for recently characterized immunological or rheumatic diseases such as the syndrome of periodic fever with aphthous stomatitis, pharyngitis, and adenitis (PFAPA) [38] or IgG4-related disease [39].

Currently, few international guidelines or consensus statements regarding steroid therapy are available. A European expert consensus statement for the diagnosis,

initiation and safety monitoring of therapeutic agents for the treatment of arthritis and systemic features. Arthritis Care Res (Hoboken) 63:465–482
37. Eleftheriou D, Levin M, Shingadia D, Tulloh R, Klein NJ, Brogan PA (2014) Management of Kawasaki disease. Arch Dis Child 99:74–83
38. Vigo G, Zulian F (2012) Periodic fevers with aphthous stomatitis, pharyngitis, and adenitis (PFAPA). Autoimmun Rev 12:52–55
39. Stone JH, Zen Y, Deshpande V (2012) IgG4-related disease. N Engl J Med 366:539–551
40. Husebye ES, Allolio B, Arlt W, Badenhoop K, Bensing S, Betterle C, Falorni A, Gan EH, Hulting AL, Kasperlik-Zaluska A, Kämpe O, Løvås K, Meyer G, Pearce SH (2014) Consensus statement on the diagnosis, treatment and follow-up of patients with primary adrenal insufficiency. J Intern Med 275:104–115
41. Hoes JN, Jacobs JW, Boers M, Boumpas D, Buttgereit F, Caeyers N, Choy EH, Cutolo M, Da Silva JA, Esselens G, Guillevin L, Hafstrom I, Kirwan JR, Rovensky J, Russell A, Saag KG, Svensson B, Westhovens R, Zeidler H, Bijlsma JW (2007) EULAR evidence-based recommendations on the management of systemic glucocorticoid therapy in rheumatic diseases. Ann Rheum Dis 66:1560–1567
42. van der Goes MC, Jacobs JW, Boers M, Andrews T, Blom-Bakkers MA, Buttgereit F, Caeyers N, Cutolo M, Da Silva JA, Guillevin L, Kirwan JR, Rovensky J, Severijns G, Webber S, Westhovens R, Bijlsma JW (2010) Monitoring adverse events of low-dose glucocorticoid therapy: EULAR recommendations for clinical trials and daily practice. Ann Rheum Dis 69:1913–1919
43. Duru N, van der Goes MC, Jacobs JW, Andrews T, Boers M, Buttgereit F, Caeyers N, Cutolo M, Halliday S, Da Silva JA, Kirwan JR, Ray D, Rovensky J, Severijns G, Westhovens R, Bijlsma JW (2013) EULAR evidence-based and consensus-based recommendations on the management of medium to high-dose glucocorticoid therapy in rheumatic diseases. Ann Rheum Dis 72:1905–1913

Corticosteroids in the Treatment of Childhood Rheumatic Diseases: A Historical Review

Ross E. Petty

Corticosteroids, in one form or another, are major components of the armamentarium the pediatric rheumatologist uses to treat many of the rheumatic diseases of childhood. Their introduction in 1949 revolutionized the pharmacologic care of adults with rheumatoid arthritis (RA), and soon thereafter, their use in observational studies of children with chronic arthritis and other rheumatic diseases was reported. That they continue to have a prominent place in treating children with rheumatic diseases is a reflection of their role as potent suppressors of inflammation (notwithstanding their significant side effects) and the fact that, until quite recently, there was little other effective treatment to offer children aside from symptomatic relief with nonsteroidal anti-inflammatory drugs. The early application of corticosteroids to the treatment of childhood rheumatic diseases is reviewed in this chapter.

The Origins of Corticosteroid Therapy

Hench and Kendall described the remarkable effects of cortisone on the inflammation of RA in a detailed account published in the *Mayo Clinic Proceedings* in 1949 [1]. For their work, Hench, a rheumatologist; Kendall, a biochemist, both at the Mayo Clinic in Rochester, Minnesota; and Reichstein, a steroid chemist in Basel, Switzerland, received the Nobel Prize in Medicine in 1950 [2].

Several apparently unrelated clinical observations led Hench to collaborate with Kendall on evaluation of the therapeutic effect of adrenocortical hormones in RA. Hench had studied the remissions in RA induced by pregnancy [3] and jaundice

R.E. Petty
Pediatric Rheumatology, University of British Columbia, British Columbia's Children's Hospital, Vancouver, Canada
e-mail: rpetty@cw.bc.ca

R. Cimaz (ed.), *Systemic Corticosteroids for Inflammatory Disorders in Pediatrics*, DOI 10.1007/978-3-319-16056-6_2

[4] and postulated that a naturally occurring factor common to both could be responsible for remissions in joint disease. Of interest, George Frederic Still had also noted marked improvement in children with chronic arthritis following "catarrhal jaundice" [5]. (Crocker and colleagues more recently argued that it is changes in lipids, rather than cortisone concentrations, occurring in both pregnancy and jaundice that are responsible for the remission in inflammatory disease [6].) Hench was aware of the brief remissions in RA induced by surgery, a procedure known to be accompanied by stimulation of the adrenal glands, and began collaborations with Kendall, who was actively investigating the many steroids found in the adrenal cortex. With the purification of sufficient quantities of one steroid, "compound E," from bovine bile, it was administered to a young woman with severe RA. The result, known to all rheumatologists, was that the patient, who had been unable to walk, resumed ambulation within days of receiving the drug. Her recovery prompted the use of compound E in 14 other patients with RA, with similar dramatic effects. Compound E was renamed cortisone. The early studies of the use of cortisone in adults with RA are thoroughly reviewed by Lundberg and colleagues [7].

Corticosteroids in the Treatment of Childhood Arthritis

Elkinton and colleagues [8] (1949) reported the use of adrenocorticotropic hormone (ACTH) in two children with juvenile rheumatoid arthritis (JRA). The clinical response was prompt, but fever and arthritis returned when the drug was discontinued. Bergman and Kinberger [9] may have been the first (1950) to report the use of a corticosteroid (desoxycorticosterone acetate) in the treatment of a child with chronic arthritis [9]. In 1951, Wolman described the striking response to oral cortisone in children with chronic arthritis, rheumatic fever, and nephrotic syndrome [10]. This detailed report also documented the disease recurrence after cortisone was discontinued, often because of unavailability of the drug.

In 1952, Bunim et al. [11] described the effects of cortisone in 31 children with active rheumatic carditis and seven children with JRA. The manifestations of active rheumatic fever responded within a few days, but relapses were noted when the cortisone dose was reduced in some patients. Barkin et al. had described the outcome in 51 children with JRA in the pre-corticosteroid era [12]; 11 of 51 patients died (eight from the effects of amyloidosis), and seven were confined to bed or wheelchair. Against this background, the effect of corticosteroids reported by Bunim et al. was dramatic: three of five children who were bed-ridden prior to treatment with cortisone and had arthritis for less than 1 year regained full joint function within 2 months; the remaining two had had arthritis for longer periods, but became ambulatory after 2 and 24 months, respectively. The authors noted that some changes (erosions, muscle wasting) were not reversible, and that relapse of active arthritis following cessation of cortisone was frequent.

This encouraging study was followed by others with inconsistent conclusions. A randomized prospective trial compared aspirin ($n = 12$) and cortisone ($n = 13$) in children with “Still's disease” [13]. Patients in each group were treated over a period of 1 year in blocks of 12 weeks followed by a 1-week period off drugs. Cortisone was given in a dose of 300 mg on the first day with a taper to 100 mg/day by 1 week (equivalent to 20 mg of prednisone or prednisolone). Aspirin was given in a dose of 6 g/day for the first week, then 2 g/day for the second week with subsequent variation in the dose between 2 and 6 g depending on clinical state. Later in the study the interrupted treatment courses were abandoned in favor of continuous treatment. At 1 year, overall improvement in both groups was similar. Glyn has written an interesting first-hand account of the early cortisone versus aspirin trials in adults in the United Kingdom [14].

Harnagel reported somewhat discouraging results in a case series of 15 children with JRA, 80 % of whom had symptomatic improvement, but only 40 % of whom had objective improvement while taking prednisone or prednisolone [15]. Harnagel noted, also, that there were frequent side effects: “moon face,” acne, striae, psychologic changes, diabetes mellitus. Lindbjerg [16] reported similarly unimpressive results in a retrospective review of children with JRA, noting that those treated with corticosteroids (usually ACTH sometimes followed by cortisone or prednisone) were no better than those treated with gold and aspirin. These early, somewhat discouraging results of corticosteroid treatment in children are not entirely explicable, although dose and duration of therapy, disease severity and type, study design, and therapeutic goal may have played a role in some instances. By contrast, Schlesinger and colleagues [17] reported the disease course and treatment in 100 children with Still's disease, and noted the marked benefit associated with cortisone treatment.

Although the literature does not document other randomized controlled trials of cortisone, ACTH, or other forms of glucocorticoids in children with chronic arthritis, these drugs became widely used. No formal dose-finding studies were reported, and regimens of administration were based on individual clinicians' experience. In the United Kingdom, in particular, alternate-day prednisone was widely used. In other parts of the world, prednisone was often administered daily, or multiple times each day. Prednisolone (in Europe) and prednisone (in North America) became the glucocorticoid drug of choice for oral administration. Prednisone is rapidly converted to its active form, prednisolone, by the liver, and in the absence of severe liver disease, the relative anti-inflammatory potency of these two drugs is equivalent.

Initially, both ACTH and cortisone were used. There was no consistent evidence that endogenous ACTH production or adrenal gland function was diminished in patients with arthritis, and it was clear that pharmacologic rather than physiologic doses of cortisone were required to suppress joint inflammation. It seemed logical to use the effective agent (cortisone) rather than ACTH, but concern about major side effects (particularly growth suppression and osteoporosis) prompted studies comparing the effects of ACTH versus prednisone on the frequency and severity of these complications. Zutshi et al. [18] concluded that ACTH may be superior to prednisolone in this regard. Ansell and Bywaters [19] reported the good effect of ACTH in six children with Still's disease and one with systemic lupus erythematosus (SLE), using a daily intramuscular administration, intermittent muscular administration, or intermittent intravenous administration.

In spite of these early observations, ACTH is no longer used to treated inflammatory disease in children for many reasons: It required intramuscular injection, it was not always readily available, was poorly standardized [18], and, in recent years, has become very expensive.

Intra-articular injection of corticosteroid has a long history in adult rheumatology [20]. However, there was concern that intra-articular corticosteroids might be harmful to the immature cartilage and it was not until the mid-1980s that injection of triamcinolone hexacetonide into inflamed joints in children with juvenile idiopathic arthritis (JIA) was demonstrated to be effective [21] and safe [22]. The superiority of triamcinolone hexacetonide has been demonstrated [23], although triamcinolone acetonide is still widely used, and for small joint or tendon sheath injections cortisone may be preferred.

For active anterior uveitis, topical corticosteroid, reported by Smiley and colleagues in 1957 [24], in an approach that remains essentially unchanged today, is usual first-line therapy, although it is frequently ineffective and it is recommended that the duration of its use be limited because of the risk of cataract and increased intraocular pressure [25]. Subconjunctival steroid injections are occasionally used.

Corticosteroids in Treatment of Connective Tissue Diseases of Childhood

The potent anti-inflammatory effects of corticosteroids in children with juvenile arthritis led to their use in children with other chronic rheumatic diseases.

Elkinton and colleagues reported (1949) the effective use of ACTH in a 6-year-old boy with dermatomyositis. Thorn and colleagues described the use of ACTH in two children with dermatomyositis [26] in 1950. Wedgwood and colleagues later evaluated the effectiveness of ACTH in these patients as equivocal [27]. Bitnum et al. noted the use of ACTH or cortisone in nine children with dermatomyositis [28]. Wedgwood et al. described the treatment of 11 children with dermatomyositis with ACTH or cortisone [27]. Seven patients received prolonged courses of ACTH (sometimes together with testosterone), and four patients received cortisone. In children with active disease, the immediate effects were very promising, but the authors noted that two of the children died subsequently. Hill and Wood [29] emphasized the import role of corticosteroids in the successful outcome of juvenile dermatomyositis. Sullivan et al. [30] documented the benefit of high-dose prednisone given up to four times daily in children with severe dermatomyositis. Prednisone remains the mainstay of the initial treatment of this disease, coupled with methotrexate.

A few months after the publication of the seminal paper by Hench et al., Harvey and colleagues [31] reported the dramatic benefit of ACTH on four adults with SLE. The first large series of children ($n = 37$) with SLE who were treated with prednisone was published by Cook et al. in 1960 [32]. Jacobs described a similar group of children with SLE in 1963, some of whom had anticonvulsant-induced disease, and noted the beneficial effect of prednisone in both groups [33]. Corticosteroids are now an essential component of the treatment of almost every child with SLE. By contrast, systemic scleroderma is corticosteroid unresponsive, although morphea or localized scleroderma is most often treated with a combination of prednisone (for a period of a few months) and methotrexate (for a longer period) [34].

Case reports and small case series of children with polyarteritis [35] and Wegener's granulomatosis [36] were reported in 1950 and 1979, respectively, and with one exception, corticosteroid treatment of systemic vasculitis became the standard of care. The controversy surrounding the use of corticosteroids in Kawasaki disease (KD), the exception, is not entirely settled. Kato et al. [37] compared the frequency of coronary artery disease in five groups of children with KD each treated with a different regimen. He and his colleagues concluded that children treated with prednisone had the highest frequency of coronary artery disease. This study had important design flaws, but had the effect of making corticosteroid therapy of KD contraindicated. In a subsequent study, Kijima and colleagues [38] demonstrated that in patients with KD and with dilated coronary arteries, intravenous pulse methylprednisolone (30 mg/kg/days × 3 days) prevented the worsening of the change or reversed the changes altogether. Corticosteroids are now considered to be second-line therapy in children who are resistant to treatment with intravenous immunoglobulin [39], and their place as first-line therapy is being investigated [40, 41].

Pursuit of Efficacy with Minimal Toxicity

Most rheumatic diseases are chronic, and require therapy over a period of years. Corticosteroids, while remarkably effective suppressors of inflammation, are the cause of considerable morbidity when given for more than a few weeks at high doses. Attempts to minimize toxicity have taken two paths. First, administration of the lowest possible effective dose for the shortest possible period is accepted practice. Administration of the drugs on an intermittent (i.e., alternate day) basis definitely diminishes side effects, but may not be as effective, especially in active or severe disease. Administration of high-dose intravenous "pulse" methylprednisolone is often favored in systemic connective tissue diseases because it minimizes the amount and duration of daily oral therapy. Cole and colleagues [42] reported the successful use of intravenous "pulse" corticosteroids in the treatment of life-threatening glomerulonephritis in eight patients, two of whom had Henoch–Schönlein purpura. Levinsky et al. [43] described the effectiveness of high-dose intravenous methylprednisolone in two patients (age 18 and 11 years) with SLE. Miller reported the successful use of large doses of corticosteroids in children with rheumatic diseases [44]. In this study, children with polyarticular JRA ($n=4$), systemic JRA ($n=5$), dermatomyositis ($n=4$), SLE ($n=2$), and other disorders received either intravenous hydrocortisone (500 mg q6h × 4 doses), or intravenous methylprednisolone (30 mg/kg) with good effect and few side effects over a follow-up period of up to 3 years. Intravenous methylprednisolone pulse therapy is now widely used in the treatment of a variety of childhood rheumatic diseases, especially systemic JIA, SLE, dermatomyositis, and many of the vasculitides.

Use of local therapy (e.g., intra-articular corticosteroids) rather than systemic corticosteroids can also minimize systemic toxicity (growth suppression, weight gain, etc.).

The second approach has been to develop corticosteroids with less toxicity. Deflazacort, a derivative of prednisolone, has been alleged to be superior to prednisone or prednisolone with regard to weight gain, growth in height, and bone mineralization, while having an equivalent anti-inflammatory effect at 6 mg compared with prednisolone at 5 mg (reviewed by Joshi and Rajeshwari) [45]. A prospective randomized trial in children with JIA confirmed a modest benefit of alternate-day low-dose deflazacort over alternate-day low-dose prednisolone with respect to bone mineralization [46]. The published literature describing the use of deflazacort in children with rheumatic diseases is very limited; it is not universally available, and its current use appears to be restricted primarily to the treatment of children with Duchenne muscular dystrophy.

Summary

The role of corticosteroids today in the management of childhood rheumatic diseases is well established. Toxicity remains a major concern and is related primarily to drug dose, frequency of drug administration, and duration of therapy. As a result, corticosteroids should be administered in the lowest effective dose, given as infrequently as possible, for as short a time period as possible. In the management of JIA, prednisone is ordinarily restricted to be used as a "bridge" while awaiting the effect of agents such as methotrexate, and in the acute management of active systemic features of systemic JIA [47]. Intra-articular triamcinolone hexacetonide has an important place in the management of arthritis. Topical corticosteroids retain a vital role in the management of uveitis. Systemic corticosteroids (oral prednisone and/or prednisolone or intravenous "pulse" methylprednisolone) are essential components of the management of SLE, dermatomyositis, and the vasculitides. The benefit of one drug (deflazacort) over others with respect to toxicity is doubtful. With the advent of the newer disease-modifying anti-inflammatory drugs and the biologics, toxicity is a lesser problem because long-term corticosteroid use is much less frequent.

References

1. Hench PS, Kendall EC (1949) The effect of a hormone of the adrenal cortex (17-hydroxy-11 dehydrocorticosterone, Compound E) and of pituitary adrenocorticotropic hormone on rheumatoid arthritis. Mayo Clin Proc 24:181–197
2. Zetterstrom R (2008) The discovery that cortisone may effectively ameliorate inflammatory and allergic disease. Acta Paediatr 97:513–517
3. Hench PS (1938) The ameliorating effect of pregnancy on chronic atrophic (infectious rheumatoid) arthritis, fibrositis and intermittent hydrarthrosis. Proc Staff Meet Mayo Clin 13:161–167

4. Hench PS (1938) Effect of spontaneous jaundice on rheumatoid (atrophic) arthritis. Brit Med J 2(4850):394–398
5. Still GF (1897) On a form of chronic joint disease in children. Med Chir Trans 80:47. Reprinted in Am J Dis Child 132(1978) 195–200
6. Crocker I, Lawson N, Fletcher J (2002) Effect of pregnancy and obstructive jaundice on inflammatory diseases: the work of PS Hench revisited. Ann Rheum Dis 61:307–310
7. Lundberg IE, Grundtman C, Larsson E, Klareskog L (2004) Corticosteroids-from an idea to clinical use. Best Pract Res Clin Rheumatol 18:7–19
8. Elkinton JR, Hunt AD, Godfrey L, McCrory WW, Rogerson AD, Stokes J (1949) Effects of pituitary adrenocorticotropic hormone (ACTH) therapy. JAMA 141:1273–1279
9. Bergman B, Kinberger FR (1950) A case report of the use of combined DOCA with ascorbic acid in a 12-year-old child with rheumatoid arthritis. J Pediatr 37:774–777
10. Wolman B (1951) The use of oral cortisone in paediatrics. Br Med J 2(4742):1246–1250
11. Bunim JJ, Kuttner AG, Baldwin JS, McEwen C (1952) Cortisone and corticotropin in rheumatic fever and juvenile rheumatoid arthritis. JAMA 150:1273–1278
12. Barkin RE (1952) Juvenile rheumatoid arthritis: a long-term followup. Ann Rheum Dis 11:316–317
13. Ansell BM, Bywaters EGL, Isdale IC (1956) Comparison of aspirin and cortisone in treatment of juvenile rheumatoid arthritis. Br Med J 1(4975):1075–1077
14. Glyn J (1998) The discovery and early use of cortisone. J R Soc Med 91:513–517
15. Harnagel EE (1959) Long-term use of prednisone and prednisolone in juvenile rheumatoid arthritis. AMA Am J Dis Child 97:426–431
16. Lindbjerg IF (1964) Juvenile rheumatoid arthritis. A follow-up of 75 cases. Arch Dis Child 39:576–583
17. Schlesinger BE, Forsyth CC, White RHR et al (1961) Observations on the clinical course and treatment of one hundred cases of Still's disease. Arch Dis Child 36:65–76
18. Zutshi DW, Friedman M, Ansell BM (1971) Corticotrophin therapy in juvenile chronic poly arthritis (Still's disease) and effect on growth. Arch Dis Child 48:584–593
19. Ansell BM, Bywaters EGL (1952) Clinical "assay" of corticotrophin. Preliminary comparison of methods. Ann Rheum Dis 11:213–218
20. Hollander JL, Brown EM Jr, Jessar RA, Brown CY (1951) Hydrocortisone and cortisone injected into arthritic joints. JAMA 147:1629–1635
21. Allen RC, Gross KR, Laxer RM et al (1986) Intraarticular triamcinolone hexacetonide in the management of chronic arthritis in children. Arthritis Rheum 29:997–1001
22. Sparling M, Malleson P, Wood B et al (1990) Radiographic follow-up of joints injected with triamcinolone hexacetonide for the management of childhood arthritis. Arthritis Rheum 33:821–826
23. Zulian F, Martini G, Gobber D et al (2004) Triamcinolone acetonide and hexacetonide intra-articular treatment of symmetrical joints in juvenile idiopathic arthritis: a double-blind trial. Rheumatology 43:1288–1291
24. Smiley WK, May E, Bywaters EGL (1957) Ocular presentations of Still's disease and their treatment. Ann Rheum Dis 16:371–383
25. Heiligenhaus A, Michels H, Schumacher C et al (2012) Evidence-based interdisciplinary guidelines for anti-inflammatory treatment of uveitis associated with juvenile idiopathic arthritis. Rheumatol Int 32:1121–1133
26. Thorn GW, Forsham PH, Frawley TF et al (1950) Clinical usefulness of ACTH and cortisone. N Engl J Med 242:865–872
27. Wedgwood RJP, Cook CD, Cohen J (1953) Dermatomyositis. Report of 26 cases in children with a discussion of endocrine therapy in 13. Pediatrics 12:447–466
28. Bitnum S, Daeschner CW Jr, Travis LB et al (1964) Dermatomyositis. J Pediatr 64:101–131
29. Hill RH, Wood WS (1970) Juvenile dermatomyositis. Can Med Assoc J 103:1152–1156
30. Sullivan DB, Cassidy JT, Petty RE, Burt A (1972) Prognosis in childhood dermatomyositis. J Pediatr 80:555–563

31. Harvey AM, Howard JE, Winkenwerder WL et al (1949) Observations on the effect of adrenocorticotrophic hormone (ACTH) on disseminated lupus erythematosus, drug hypersensitivity reactions and chronic bronchial asthma. Trans Am Clin Climatol Assoc 61:221–228
32. Cook CD, Wedgwood RJP, Craig JM, Hartmann JR, Janeway CA (1960) Systemic lupus erythematosus. Description of 37 cases in children and a discussion of endocrine therapy in 32 of the cases. Pediatrics 26:570–585
33. Jacobs JC (1963) Systemic lupus erythematosus in childhood. Report of thirty-five cases with discussion of seven apparently induced by anticonvulsant medication and of prognosis and treatment. Pediatrics 32:257–264
34. Uziel Y, Feldman BM, Krafchik BR et al (2000) Methotrexate and corticosteroid therapy for pediatric localized scleroderma. J Pediatr 136:91–95
35. Carey RA, Harvey AM, Howard JE (1950) The effect of adrenocorticotropic hormone (ACTH) and cortisone on the course of disseminated lupus erythematosus and periarteritis nodosa. Bull Johns Hopkins Hosp 27:427–460
36. Backman A, Grahne P, Holopainen E et al (1979) Wegener's granulomotosis in childhood. A clinical report based on 3 cases. Int J Pediatr Otorhinolaryngol 1:145–149
37. Kato H, Koito S, Yokoyama T (1979) Kawasaki disease: effect of treatment on coronary involvement. Pediatrics 63:175–179
38. Kijima Y, Kamiya T, Suzuki A et al (1982) A trial procedure to prevent aneurysm formation of the coronary arteries by steroid pulse therapy in Kawasaki disease. Jpn Circ J 46:1239–1242
39. Koboyashi T, Koboyashi T, Morikawa A et al (2013) Efficacy of intravenous immunoglobulin combined with prednisolone following resistance to initial immunoglobulin treatment of acute Kawasaki disease. J Pediatr 163:521–526
40. Inoue Y, Okada Y, Shinohara M et al (2006) A multicenter prospective randomized trial of corticosteroids in primary therapy for Kawasaki disease: clinical course and coronary artery outcome. J Pediatr 149:336–341
41. Newburger JW, Sleeper LA, McCrindle BW et al (2007) Randomized trial of pulsed corticosteroid therapy for primary treatment of Kawasaki disease. N Engl J Med 356:663–675
42. Cole BR, Brocklebank JT, Kienstra RA, Kissane JM (1976) "Pulse" methylprednisolone therapy in the treatment of severe glomerulonephritis. J Pediatr 88:307–314
43. Levinsky RJ, Cameron JS, Soothill JF (1977) Serum immune complexes and disease activity in lupus nephritis. Lancet 1(8011):564–567
44. Miller JJ III (1980) Prolonged use of large intravenous steroid pulses in the rheumatic diseases of children. Pediatrics 65:989–994
45. Joshi N, Rajeshwari K (2009) Deflazacort. J Postgrad Med 55:296–300
46. Loftus J, Allen R, Hesp R et al (1991) Randomized double-blind trial of deflazacort versus prednisone in juvenile chronic (or rheumatoid) arthritis: a relatively bone-sparing effect of deflazacort. Pediatrics 88:428–436
47. Beukelman T, Patkar NM, Saag KG et al (2011) 2011 American College of Rheumatology recommendations for the treatment of juvenile idiopathic arthritis: initiation and safety monitoring of agents for the treatment of arthritis and systemic features. Arthritis Care Res 63:465–482

Systemic Corticosteroids for Autoimmune/ Inflammatory Disorders in Children: Clinical Aspects

Pascal Pillet

Introduction

Glucocorticoids (GCs) are a class of steroid hormones released from the adrenal cortex, and their plasma concentration is controlled by the hypothalamic–pituitary–adrenal axis. Endogenous GCs affect biological processes including growth, metabolism, development, immune function, and stress response. GCs and the derived drugs (named corticosteroids) are widely used as pharmacological agents for the treatment of inflammatory disease, asthma, and immune/rheumatologic diseases. This chapter describes the mechanisms of action of synthetic GCs, prescription methods in immune/rheumatologic diseases, and the management of side effects.

Mechanisms of Action

"Corticosteroids" (GCs and mineralocorticoids) have anti-inflammatory, immunosuppressive, and cytotoxic properties. The anti-inflammatory activity of GCs is higher than natural hormones for a reduced mineralocorticoid activity. The therapeutic effects result from a genomic mechanism calling action from the GC receptor (increased synthesis of anti-inflammatory proteins, decreased synthesis and decreased half-life of RNA messengers coding for inflammatory proteins) and a nongenomic (quick) mechanism with no interaction with a surface receiver that would affect intracellular signal channels (mitogen-activated protein kinases channels, calcium fluxes). This results in a decreased production of proinflammatory

P. Pillet
Pediatric Department, Pellegrin-Enfants Hospital,
Place Amélie raba Léon, Bordeaux 33076, France
e-mail: Pascal.pillet@chu-bordeaux.fr

R. Cimaz (ed.), *Systemic Corticosteroids for Inflammatory Disorders in Pediatrics*, DOI 10.1007/978-3-319-16056-6_3

Table 1 Main molecules: comparison of corticosteroid activity

DCI	Anti-inflammatory activity	Mineralocorticoid effect	Dose equivalence (mg)	Half-life (h)
Hydrocortisone	1	1	20	8–12
Cortisone	1	0.8	25	8–12
Prednisone	4	0.8	5	12–36
Prednisolone	4	0.8	5	12–36
Methylprednisolone	5	0.5	4	12–36
Betamethasone	25–30	0	0.75	36–54
Triamcinolone	5	0	4	

cytokines and chemotactic factors as well as of intercellular adhesion molecules (ICAM-1), inhibition of the differentiation and function of macrophages, synthesis of the prostaglandins and leukotrienes, and production of free radicals. GCs also have important effects on immune response (antigen presentation, lymphocyte proliferation and differentiation) and on apoptosis.

Pharmacology

The structure of prednisolone, a reference GC, is comparable to that of natural hormone, since only a double bond differentiates them. This double bond causes an increase in anti-inflammatory activity and in plasma half-life and a decrease in the mineralocorticoid effect. Prednisone is quickly absorbed in the jejunum and is then converted into prednisolone, an active metabolite, through hepatic 11β-hydroxylation. The plasma concentration peak is obtained within 1–2 h, slows down after meals, and varies according to the type of GC. Plasma cortisol is strongly bound to cortisol-binding globulin and albumin. The binding kinetics is not linear or dose-related, and the clearance is urinary. Natural GCs follow a circadian rhythm of maximum secretion between 6 and 9 P.M. and a minimum secretion around midnight. Therefore, the administration schedule of GCs has an essential influence over pituitary secretion: A dose administered in the morning has a minimum effect, contrary to a dose taken in the evening (Table 1).

Conditions of Prescription and Main Indications (Table 2)

The prescription of GCs over a long period is an important decision in terms of consequences, considering the risks of a diagnostic error (i.e., prescription in case of infections or neoplasia) and inappropriate or delayed initiation that could impact vital or functional prognosis. The effect is suspensive, which exposes patients to quick relapses when interruptions are attempted. The side effects of GCs represent

Table 2 Main indications of corticotherapy for child inflammatory diseases

Disease type	Etiology	Remarks
Rheumatology, systemic disease	Juvenile idiopathic arthritis (JIA)	*Systemic-onset JIA*, macrophage activation syndrome, *uveitis, polyarticular JIA*
	Acute rheumatic fever	
	Juvenile dermatomyositis	
	Systemic lupus erythematosus	Pulse therapy: cardiac, nephrologic, neurological form
	Scleroderma	
	Sarcoidosis	
	Systemic vasculitis, refractory Kawasaki disease, complications of Henoch–Schönlein purpura	
Autoinflammatory	PFAPA syndrome	Treatment of crisis
Digestive	Inflammatory bowel disease, autoimmune hepatitis	
Hematological	Thrombocytopenic purpura, autoimmune hemolytic anemia	
Nephrologic	Nephrotic syndrome, glomerulonephritis	
Neurological	Systemic sclerosis, inflammatory demyelinating polyradiculoneuropathy	
Ophthalmological	*Uveitis*	

PFAPA periodic fever, aphthous stomatitis, pharyngitis, adenitis

a major worry, which justifies their use only after a definitive diagnosis has been made. According to the indication, prescription can be short or long term, preferably orally administered prednisone or prednisolone and sometimes with intravenous boluses [1]. Short treatments last less than 10 days and typically aim for an anti-inflammatory effect with high doses (2 mg/kg/day). Examples of such treatment are complicated Henoch–Schönlein purpura, Kawasaki syndrome resistant to immunoglobulins, and idiopathic thrombocytopenic purpura. Long-term treatments aim for lower doses (maximum 60–80 mg/day), with a quick taper. The initial dosing, preferably in the morning, is generally maintained 2–4 weeks, and carefully tapered in gradual steps from 1 to 4 weeks, depending on the pathology, the protocol, and the initial response. This decrease will occur faster for dosages higher than 1 mg/kg/day, with the objective of reaching a maintenance dose of 0.5 mg/kg/day and then the minimal effective dose or the discontinuation. Alternate-day dosing as used for nephrotic syndrome may attenuate the effects on growth but in other indications represents a risk of disease flare. GCs should never be interrupted abruptly, since the risk of adrenal insufficiency must be considered when the administered dose is greater than the replacement dose and when treatment exceeds 15 days. High-dosage "pulse" therapy allows one to obtain a quick anti-inflammatory effect, possibly with a corticosteroid-sparing effect. Intravenous boluses are usually recommended daily over 3 consecutive days, particularly in critical situations regarding vital or functional prognosis (severe organ involvement, hemophagocytosis, resistant Kawasaki disease). Methylprednisolone is given via an intravenous route at a dose of 30 mg/kg (max. 1 g) over a period of at least 4 h and while carefully monitoring vital signs. Intra-articular injections can be part of the therapeutic strategy for juvenile arthritis. Triamcinolone hexacetonide is the most used form because of its long-lasting effect [2].

How to Limit the Main Side Effects of GCs

GCs possess several endocrinological properties, being involved in many physiological and pathological processes; their efficacy in improving inflammatory disorders results from the pleiotropic effects of the GC receptors on multiple signaling pathways. Adverse effects include growth retardation, immunosuppression, hypertension, hyperglycemia, inhibition of wound repair, deleterious effects on bone and cartilage, metabolic disturbances (lipid and protein metabolism, muscle wasting), hydro-electrolytic imbalance, gastritis, premature atherosclerosis, and ocular (glaucoma and cataract) and dermatologic (acne, alopecia, hypertrichosis, stretch marks) complications.

Metabolic Complications

The prevention of metabolic complications (carbohydrate intolerance, hypertriglyceridemia, adiposity, protein hypercatabolism) mainly includes a dietary plan based on a hypocaloric, hyperproteic, low-salt regimen, free from quick-absorption sugars and prepared as menus adapted to the energy requirements and food habits of children.

Osteoporosis

GC-induced osteoporosis (GIO) is the most common form of iatrogenic osteoporosis and one of the most common forms of secondary osteoporosis. Fracture risk increases markedly in the first 3 months after GC initiation and decreases after discontinuation, but the risk does not return to baseline. GCs adversely affect bone strength/quality in a number of ways: They induce an imbalance between bone formation and resorption, with short- (demineralization) and long-term consequences. They inhibit bone formation (by increased apoptosis of osteoblasts and osteocytes, decreased osteoblastogenesis, and disruption of bone remodeling regulation) and they increase bone resorption (by enhanced osteoclast survival and osteoclastogenesis). Moreover, they decrease intestinal calcium absorption and increase urinary calcium excretion. Thus, GCs decrease bone mass (12 % for the first 3 months, then 3 %/year) and increase the fracture risk mainly of vertebrae [3, 4]. Prevention of osteoporosis consists in controlling the underlying inflammatory disease, sparing corticosteroid dosage, promoting physical activities, and recommending calcium intake in relation to the patient's age. In case of insufficiency, the addition of a calcium supplement at doses between 300 (<5 years) and 500 mg/day (>5 years) is important. Vitamin D supplementation, as a daily (400 UI/day at least) or quarterly (80,000 or 100,000 UI) recommendation, has the objective of obtaining a serum level of 25-OH-D3 between 20 and 40 ng/ml. Beyond 3 months of corticosteroid treatment, it is advisable to perform a reference densitometry (DXA) and monitor the Z score according to its initial value, the status of inflammatory disease, and the dose and duration of GC therapy. An evaluation of bone density and metabolism can be typically proposed in severe cases once to twice a year. The use of bisphosphonate therapy for children is still under discussion. It is recommended only after specialized advice in cases of fractures, bone pain, or quick degradation of bone density.

Growth-Retarding Effects

A growth delay is unavoidable beyond 0.3 mg/kg/day (resistance to growth hormone, decrease of growth hormone and insulin-like growth factor-1, serum levels, action on growth plate). Other factors, for example, inflammatory and nutritional factors, also play a role. In some situations, growth hormone treatment may be discussed [5].

Infections

The risk for community-based and/or opportunistic infections is very high at dosages exceeding 2 mg/kg/day for more than 15 days, or after repeated intravenous boluses. However, other predisposing factors such as the inflammatory disease, malnutrition, hyperglycemia, and concomitant immunosuppressors should be considered. It is advisable to inform patients and their families about the need for an early consultation in case of fever, about environmental risks (e.g., unpasteurized foods, uncooked meats), contact with animals, and travels to endemic areas for unusual pathogens such as histoplasmosis. Observance of the immunization schedule is essential, and flu vaccines and pneumococcal vaccines are especially recommended. Live vaccines are contraindicated while on chronic corticosteroid treatment. Continuous trimethoprim-sulfamethoxazole may be recommended as a prevention of *Pneumocystis jirovecii* infection. Herpes virus infections warrant early treatment with acyclovir. Contact with varicella for a high-risk child requires administration within 4 days of specific anti-VZV immunoglobulins, which is the most commonly recommended approach. If not possible, chemoprophylaxis with acyclovir (80 mg/kg/day, divided into four doses, for 7 days) starting between the seventh and tenth day after the exposure should be proposed.

Psychiatric Disturbances

GCs are mediators of stress response. Steroid receptors are expressed in different areas of the brain and their role is related to the regulation of various neurotransmitters, including serotonin and dopamine. In particular, in the central nervous system, GCs exert their potential effects at the hippocampal level, a structure intimately involved in the limbic system, which provides the processing of emotional information and memory. Behavioral changes and mood disorders (irritability, agitation, anxiety, insomnia, and depression) are frequent and difficult to predict and sometimes to distinguish from symptoms related to the underlying illness [6]. Increased appetite with a resulting increase of body weight is frequent. Psychotic conditions (mania, psychosis, and delirium), nearly always transient, have been described but remain rare. Sleep disorders can be limited by administration of GCs in the morning.

Conclusion

In recent years, patient management for inflammatory diseases has seen considerable improvements due to new and effective therapies. However, GCs still remain the reference treatment for many disorders. The administration of GCs is an important decision, which should be taken within a precise treatment plan and with clear objectives. Parents and families should be informed of this plan and of the possible risks and benefits. We should always aim to find a balance between sufficient anti-inflammatory activity and acceptable undesired effects, which must be monitored and prevented when possible.

References

1. Bader-Meunier B (2001) Comment prescrire les corticoïdes systémiques ? In: Dommergues JP (ed) Corticotherapie chez l'enfant. Progrès en Pédiatrie, Doin (ed), Rueil Malmaison, France pp 31–34
2. Cattalini M, Maduskuie V, Fawcett PT et al (2008) Predicting duration of beneficial effect of joint injection among children with chronic arthritis by measuring biomarkers concentration in synovial fluid at the time of injection. Clin Exp Rheumatol 26(6):1153–1160
3. Olney RC (2009) Mechanisms of impaired growth: effect of steroids on bone and cartilage. Horm Res 72(Suppl 1):30–35. Epub 2009 Nov 27. Review
4. Huber AM, Gaboury I, Cabral DA et al; Canadian Steroid-Associated Osteoporosis in the Pediatric Population (STOPP) Consortium (2010) Prevalent vertebral fractures among children initiating glucocorticoid therapy for the treatment of rheumatic disorders. Arthritis Care Res (Hoboken) 62(4):516–526
5. Bechtold S, Dalla Pozza R, Schwarz HP, Simon D (2009) Effects of growth hormone treatment in juvenile idiopathic arthritis: bone and body composition. Horm Res 72(Suppl 1):60–64. Review
6. Ciriaco M, Ventrice P, Russo G, Scicchitano M, Mazzitello G, Scicchitano F, Russo E (2013) Corticosteroid-related central nervous system side effects. J Pharmacol Pharmacother 4(Suppl 1): S94–S98

The Molecular and Cellular Mechanisms Responsible for the Anti-inflammatory and Immunosuppressive Effects of Glucocorticoids

Giuseppe Nocentini, Graziella Migliorati, and Carlo Riccardi

Introduction

Owing to their powerful anti-inflammatory and immunomodulatory actions, glucocorticoids (GCs) are widely used to treat both acute and chronic inflammatory conditions. GCs also induce immunosuppression and therefore are administered after organ transplantation, during severe allergic reactions or autoimmune flare-ups, and as part of chemotherapy regimens. However, long-term and intense stimulation of GC receptors (GRs) causes adverse effects that are collectively termed Cushing's syndrome.

During the past century, researchers have produced more potent GCs that have longer half-lives and lack virtually all of the mineral corticoid effects (e.g., betamethasone and dexamethasone) compared with endogenous GC (cortisol) and the first synthetic GC (prednisolone).

Molecules that have entered the clinic in the past 20 years are GC analogues that decrease the risk-to-benefit ratios for the long-term topical treatment of some diseases. These molecules have improved pharmacokinetic properties and have increased the desired effects in peripheral tissues while simultaneously decreasing the unwanted systemic effects. However, it seems they have a mechanism of action identical to that of older GCs. In this chapter, we present the molecular and cellular mechanisms responsible for the powerful anti-inflammatory and immunosuppressive effects of GCs.

G. Nocentini • G. Migliorati • C. Riccardi (✉)
Section of Pharmacology, Department of Medicine, University of Perugia, Building D, 2nd floor, Severi Square 1, San Sisto, Perugia I-06132, Italy
e-mail: giuseppe.nocentini@unipg.it

R. Cimaz (ed.), *Systemic Corticosteroids for Inflammatory Disorders in Pediatrics*, DOI 10.1007/978-3-319-16056-6_4

Molecular Mechanisms of Glucocorticoids

GCs exert different effects in different tissues. For example, GCs can trigger apoptosis in some lymphocytes but protect against cell death in other lymphocytes or parenchymal cells in inflamed tissues. Array studies evaluating the messenger RNA (mRNA) levels from a diverse cell population demonstrated that these differences are because the majority of genes modulated by GCs in a certain cell type are not expressed in cells with other phenotypes. In the following paragraphs, we explain how it is possible that a drug that targets just one receptor causes this amazing variety by both genomic and nongenomic effects, as summarized in Fig. 1.

Genomic Effects

Owing to their hydrophobic nature, GCs pass from the circulation into cells where they bind the ubiquitously expressed GC receptor (GR). GR is located in the cytoplasm where it exists in a multimeric chaperone complex composed of heat shock proteins (HSP90AA1 and HSP70), HSP-binding phosphoprotein p23, immunophilins (FKBP51, FKBP52, Cyp44, and PP5), Hip, Hop, and other factors [76, 100]. The chaperone heat shock protein 90 kDa alpha, class A member 1 (HSP90AA1), maintains GR in a favorable conformational state that is required for high-affinity ligand binding and cytoplasmic retention.

There are two main isoforms of human GR (hGR), the predominant hGRα and hGRβ. Each of the GR mRNA species, α and β, produces at least eight functional GR N-terminal isoforms via translational modifications, each with potentially unique transcriptional activities [79]. For example, the GRα isoforms, GR-A, GR-B, and GR-C, induce Jurkat cell apoptosis, whereas the GR-D isoform does not [103]. Moreover, GRs can be phosphorylated and sumoylated, thereby modulating their function and half-life [15, 79]. hGRβ is unable to bind any GCs and is transcriptionally inactive; thus, it acts as a dominant-negative regulator of hGRα [69].

Upon GC binding, GRα changes conformation and owing to the chaperone machinery, the receptor translocates to the nucleus [100] to positively and negatively regulate gene transcription.

Upregulation of Gene Transcription

The primary manner by which activated GRα (herein referred to as GR) upregulates gene transcription (also known as transactivation) is via dimerization and binding to GC-response elements (GREs) that are present in one or more copies in the promoter regions of hundreds of genes. In some cases, the GRE is far from the transcriptional start site. Although the canonical GRE was defined as the palindromic sequence A-G-A-A-C-A-N-N-N-T-G-T-T-C-T (where N indicates any nucleotide),

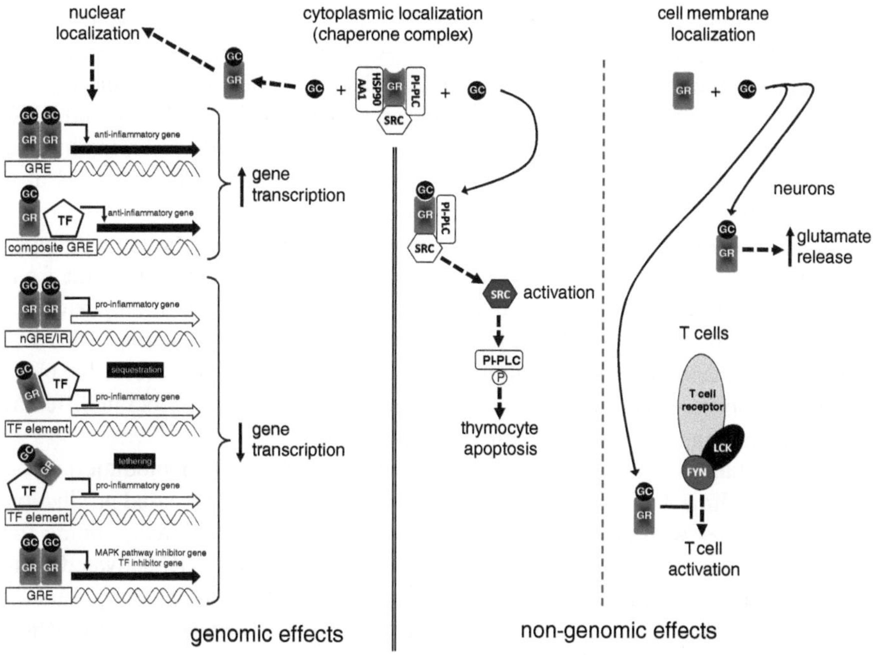

Fig. 1 Mechanism of action of glucocorticoids. Glucocorticoids (*GCs*) act through two mechanisms: genomic (main mechanism) and nongenomic (accessory but immediately effective). GCs pass from the circulation into cells where they bind GC receptor (*GR*), located in a cytoplasmic chaperone complex (*middle*), in complexes located in the cell membranes (*right*) or in other cellular structures (not shown). The chaperone complex is formed by several proteins including heat shock protein 90 kDa alpha, class A member 1 (*HSP90AA1*), phosphatidylinositol-specific phospholipase C (*PI-PLC*) and SRC proto-oncogene, nonreceptor tyrosine kinase (*SRC*). Following nuclear translocation of activated GR (*left*), genomic effects are exerted by at least six mechanisms: (1) upregulation of gene transcription by binding GC-response elements (*GRE*); (2) upregulation of gene transcription by activation of transcription factors (*TF*) that bind DNA next to a GR-binding element (composite GRE); (3) downregulation of gene transcription by binding negative GRE (*nGRE*) characterized by inverted repeat (*IR*); (4) downregulation of gene transcription by binding TFs and inhibiting their binding to DNA (sequestration); (5) downregulation of gene transcription by binding TFs and inhibiting their transcriptional activity (tethering); (6) upregulation of gene transcription by binding GRE in the promoter region of genes coding for inhibitors of TF (conclusively leading to downregulation of gene transcription) or proinflammatory pathways, such as the MAPK pathway. Nongenomic effects depend on the localization of GR and the GR-bound proteins. In thymocytes, activated GR activates SRC that, in turn, phosphorylates PI-PLC, leading to thymocyte apoptosis. In neurons of the prefrontal and frontal cortex, GR is present is synaptosomes and in presynaptic spines and its activation increases the readily releasable pool of glutamate vesicles. In T cells, GR is close to T cell receptor (TCR) complex and GR activation inhibits TCR-dependent activation of lymphocyte-specific protein tyrosine kinase (LCK) and FYN oncogene related to SRC, FGR, and YES (FYN), inhibiting T cell activation

many variations are possible, particularly in the 3′ half site. The variations are described by the sequence N-G-N-(A,T)-C-(A,G,T)-N-N-N-(A,T)-G-T-(C,T)-C-T [98]. The interaction between GR and DNA induces a variety of coregulatory factors – including Brg1, histone acetyl transferases such as CBP or SRC-1, and RNA polymerase II – to physically associate with GR, be recruited to chromatin, and ultimately drive transcription [17]. In this context, the cellular effects of GR also depend on the types and expression levels of coactivators.

In the promoters of some genes, GR monomers or dimers collaborate with other transcription factors to cooperatively enhance transcription. This can result from GR and other transcription factors binding to adjacent binding sites (composite elements) or from GR binding DNA-bound transcription factors (tethering) [60, 89]. The gene transcription effects occur in chromatin where the DNA is accessible independent of hormone action [46], thus modulating distinct genomic loci in different cells and resulting in tissue- and cell-specific effects.

Several, but not all, metabolic effects of GC depend on GR homodimerization and GRE binding. The same mechanism is responsible for the increased production of several genes with anti-inflammatory or immunosuppressive effects coding for inhibitors of proinflammatory cytoplasmic pathways (section "GC-activated anti-inflammatory and immunosuppressive pathways"), modulators of transcription factors (section "Downregulation of gene transcription by GR-dependent upregulation of inhibitory factors"), and other proteins such as tristetraprolin (TTP), a protein favoring destabilization and degradation of mRNAs coding for proinflammatory factors [86].

Downregulation of Gene Transcription

GR predominantly downregulates gene transcription of cytokines and other factors that contribute to the development of inflammation and immune response by inhibiting protein-to-protein interactions (also known as sequestration). This signaling mechanism is best characterized for the inhibition of transcription factors nuclear factor κB (NF-κB), activator protein-1 (AP-1), nuclear factor of activated T-cells and Smad3 [31]. For example, NF-κB is maintained in an inactive state via interaction with its inhibitor IκB. NF-κB is activated by proinflammatory stimuli, which causes IκB to be phosphorylated and dissociate from the IκB/NF-κB complex. GR can repress NF-κB-mediated gene activation by physically interacting with the p65 subunit of NF-κB, thereby sequestering p65 [58].

GR can also inhibit transcription factors such as NF-κB by forming a complex when they are bound to DNA and preventing the recruitment of transcriptional machinery (effect also known as tethering) [14]. The sequestration mechanism of GR action affects the activity of transcription factors expressed in the cell, causing tissue- and cell-specific effects.

In the promoter of genes that are downregulated by GC, the sequence C-T-C-C-$(N)_{0-2}$-G-G-A-G-A has been described [92]. This sequence is suggested to represent a DNA-binding site called simple negative GRE (nGRE) or inverted repeat (IR) to which the GR homodimer binds. nGREs mediate transrepression by direct binding of activated GR that assembles a repressing complex. In other genes, nGREs are located close to DNA-binding sites for other transcription factors. Thus, GR inhibits transcription factor activity by competing with and displacing transcription factors from DNA [36]. For example, GR binding to the nGRE in the promoter of hFas ligand prevents NF-κB binding and inhibits Fas ligand expression [67]. In other cases, GR binding to the GRE or nGRE inhibits transcription factor binding to a DNA-binding site proximal to the GR binding site (so-called composite elements) [14].

Downregulation of Gene Transcription by GR-Dependent Upregulation of Inhibitory Factors

One mechanism that explains the powerful anti-inflammatory effects of GC is the very rapid, GRE-dependent upregulation of proteins that inhibit transcription factors. Among these proteins, glucocorticoid-induced leucine zipper (GILZ), IκB (an inhibitor of NF-κB) [5], and Krüppel-like factor 2 (KLF2; an inhibitor of NF-κB and AP-1) [30] are the best characterized.

GILZ was originally identified in 1997 during a systematic study of genes transcriptionally induced by GC [28]. It is one of the few genes induced by GC in nearly all immune cell types. The finding that *GILZ* silencing abrogates DEX antiproliferative activity [9] and reduces GC-mediated inhibition of cytokine-induced cyclooxygenase (COX)-2 expression [104] distinguished *GILZ* as a critical mediator of GC effects. GILZ overexpression modulates several cellular pathways [8]; however, it primarily inhibits transcription factors such as NF-κB and AP-1 [7, 34, 35, 61].

In addition to the GC-dependent effects on transcription factor modulators, which seem to be very rapid (of the order of hours), GR-dependent direct and indirect modulation of several transcription factors causes a striking amplification effect. This results in the modulation of thousands of genes in the subsequent days following GC treatment [22].

Nongenomic Effects

Although most GC immunosuppressive and anti-inflammatory effects are mediated through genomic effects that require hours to days, others take place within minutes (e.g., rapid cardiovascular protective effects, rapid clinical improvement of anaphylactic reactions, and effects on glutamate and GABA release). These cannot be explained by genomic mechanisms. Several hypotheses have been suggested to explain these effects, including aspecific effects on cell membrane fluidity or activation of G protein-coupled receptors specific for GCs [53, 93]. Although it is increasingly recognized that receptors activated by GCs are present in the plasma membrane and are capable of activating cytoplasmic pathways, a transmembrane receptor specific for GCs has not yet been described. By contrast, recent studies suggest that GC-free GRs are not confined to the GR chaperone complex but rather are present in other cellular locations, including the cell membrane [70], likely in association with other receptors or signaling molecules. In this case, GRα activation by GC promotes not only the activation of GRα but also of the other receptors/signaling molecules [90].

Indeed, several studies suggest that the nongenomic effects of GR depend on the particular localization of GR in cells. For example, in adenocarcinoma cells, GR binds proto-oncogene, nonreceptor tyrosine kinase (SRC) and activated GR releases SRC, which subsequently phosphorylates annexin-1. Phosphorylated annexin-1, in turn, displaces the adaptor protein Grb2 from epidermal growth factor receptor. Consequently, GR activation inhibits epidermal growth factor receptor-dependent activation of PLA2 and arachidonic acid release [27]. In thymocytes, GR binds phosphatidylinositol-specific phospholipase C and SRC, and activated GR determines the rapid phosphorylation and activation of phosphatidylinositol-specific phospholipase C due to SRC, which ultimately leads to thymocyte apoptosis [55]. In T cells, GR has a close physical and functional interaction with the T cell receptor (TCR) complex, and GR activation causes a rapid dissolution of TCR-linked GR complexes and inhibits Lck and Fyn, kinases immediately downstream of the TCR [52]. In neurons of the prefrontal and frontal cortex, GR is present in synaptosomes, as well as in presynaptic membranes and postsynaptic spines, and its activation increases the readily releasable pool of glutamate vesicles in synaptic terminals [95].

When considering the effects of GC on the central nervous system, it should be noted that neurosteroids (e.g., allopregnanolone and tetrahydrodeoxycorticosterone) target $GABA_A$ receptors, thereby potentiating $GABA_A$ receptor-mediated currents [88]. Although it has been shown that neurosteroid levels depend on local de novo synthesis and progesterone metabolism, the potential effects of GCs on neurosteroid production cannot be ruled out.

In conclusion, the nongenomic effects of GCs result from the binding of GRs located in the cell membrane (or other cellular structures) and the consequent activation of cytoplasmic pathways not involved in gene transcription.

GC-Activated Anti-inflammatory and Immunosuppressive Pathways

Virtually all cells of the adaptive and innate immune systems are modulated by GCs. The various mechanisms include inhibiting production of a large number of proinflammatory factors that are crucial for the development, maintenance, and outcome of inflammation and autoimmune diseases. This is the primary reason why GCs remain the most potent immunosuppressive drugs available. However, GCs modulate the functions of other cells and tissues, thus causing adverse effects during long-term treatment.

Although we will focus on effects of GCs at therapeutic doses, it is interesting to note that GCs at low concentrations, particularly endogenous GCs, favor maturation and differentiation of the immune system and other tissues, including muscles and the central nervous system. Thus, it is possible that GCs determine opposing effects (e.g., apoptosis and protection against apoptosis) [16] depending on their concentration as well as the functional status of the cell.

The anti-inflammatory and immunosuppressive effects of GCs have been attributed to their ability to inhibit the activity of the transcription factors, including NF-κB, AP-1, CREB, NF-AT, STAT, IRF3, and T-bet. These transcription factors are involved in the expression of many proinflammatory genes, including the cytokines interleukin (IL)-6, IL-1β, and tumor necrosis factor-α, the chemokines macrophage inflammatory protein and RANTES, the enzymes inducible nitric oxide synthase and COX-2, and the adhesion molecules intercellular adhesion molecule-1 (ICAM-1), vascular cell adhesion molecule-1 (VCAM-1), and E-selectin [21, 32, 50, 101].

GC-induced upregulation of anti-inflammatory genes plays a key role in their anti-inflammatory and immunosuppressive activity via several mechanisms including: (1) mitogen-activated protein kinase (MAPK) pathway inhibition (upregulation of dual-specificity phosphatase-1, docking protein-1, and GILZ); (2) prostaglandin synthesis inhibition [upregulation of annexin-1 and Clara cell 10 kDa (CC10)]; (3) inhibition of T cell activation [upregulation of Src-like adaptor protein (SLAP), IL-10, and IL-1 receptor antagonist], and (4) activation of regulatory T cells [upregulation of Forkhead box P3 (FoxP3) and IL-10].

Some of the upregulated genes have multiple concurrent functions. For example, GILZ binds and inhibits NF-κB and AP-1, as well as Ras and Raf, resulting in inhibition of both the Akt and ERK pathways, two MAPK pathways that contribute to the regulation of proinflammatory transcription factors and perpetuate inflammatory cascade activation [8–10]. GC-induced annexin-1 upregulation participates in the inhibition of phospholipase A2, an enzyme that initiates the cascade leading to prostaglandin production, inhibition of tumor necrosis factor-α upregulation, and induction of IL-10, an anti-inflammatory cytokine [38, 87]. Moreover, annexin-1 inhibits MAPK signaling, either directly by regulating components of the signaling cascade or indirectly by modulating other GC-induced proteins, such as GILZ [6].

Another mechanism by which GCs regulate inflammatory processes is through modulation of the expression and activity of a variety of kinases and phosphatases [14]. For example, GC upregulates expression of dual-specificity phosphatase-1, which is a negative feedback regulator of MAPK signaling [84].

GCs activate various pathways to inhibit cell growth and induce apoptosis. Thymocytes, particularly $CD4^{+}CD8^{+}$ double-positive thymocytes, are considered the prototype of GC-induced apoptosis because of their high sensitivity to GCs. In the past, several groups (including ours) attempted to find the crucial proapoptotic event(s) – including increased or decreased gene expression – that are definitively responsible for GC-induced apoptosis. Array studies indicate that several genes that participate in different cellular functions are modulated by GC treatment, causing an imbalance between pro- and antiapoptotic genes and thus inducing apoptosis (termed the network hypothesis) [16, 83]. The dysregulated genes include genes that control the redox status and the mitochondrial machinery (including Bcl-2, Bcl-X, and Bim), as well as the Tis11 family, which is involved in mRNA stability, and the ceramide pathway [16, 71]. Other genomic and nongenomic mechanisms participate in the induction of thymocyte apoptosis, such as Src kinase activation, GILZ upregulation, or plasma membrane potential modulation, and involve aSMase, caspases-3, -8, and -9, proteasomal degradation, and lysosomal pathways [26, 54, 55]. Even mature T cells can undergo GC-mediated apoptosis [105]. Apoptosis of leukemic cells is mediated by both genomic and nongenomic mechanisms. The nongenomic mechanism involves translocation of GRs to the mitochondria upon GC binding, thereby modifying their transmembrane potential [85].

Other GC-modulated genes inhibit apoptosis, such as inhibition of activation-induced cell death (AICD) in mature T cells, whose GC-dependent reduction of CD95L transcription is one of the involved mechanisms [13]. The antiapoptotic effects of GCs are observed in several parenchymal cell types, including endometrial cells and neurons, saving peripheral tissues and contributing to the anti-inflammatory effects of GCs [45, 72].

Effects on T Lymphocytes

Recent evidence suggests that both thymic regulatory T cells (tTregs) and peripheral regulatory T cells (pTreg) are needed to establish and maintain tolerance [42]. In autoimmune diseases, several reports have demonstrated decreased numbers of Tregs or defects in Treg suppressive activity, which is either intrinsic or due to partial resistance of activated effector T cells [40, 48, 94]. Moreover, Treg expansion has been described in patients with a milder autoimmune disease as compared with patients with more aggressive disease [2, 66]. T helper (Th) 1 cells are the predominant subpopulation involved in autoimmune pathogenesis, and their secreted cytokines, IL-2 and interferon-γ, contribute to the proinflammatory phenotype. Th17 cells enhance autoimmune response progression and can drive the autoimmune response in the absence of a concomitant Th1 response [1, 18, 29].

GC treatment has several effects on T cell subsets, including Treg expansion and Th polarization. Additionally, when treating infants, the effects of GC on thymocyte maturation must also be considered.

Effects on Regulatory T Cells

In experimental models, GCs increase the frequency of Tregs, suggesting that GC-mediated immune suppression is partially achieved through increased Treg cell number or activity [24]. Clinical studies have reported a GC-dependent increase in Treg-related cytokine expression or Treg cell number and function. In patients with asthma, GC treatment induces IL-10 synthesis, a major anti-inflammatory cytokine produced by Tregs, as well as expression of the Forkhead box P3 transcription factor (FoxP3), which is typically expressed by these cells [47]. In patients with

Graves' disease, Treg cell functionality improved after dexamethasone treatment; however, their proportion remained unchanged [44]. Treg expansion has been observed in GC-treated patients with multiple sclerosis and rheumatic disease [3, 19, 33]. Finally, GC treatment increased Treg cell number in patients with systemic lupus erythematosus (SLE) [11, 91].

There is likely more than one mechanism involved in the GC-mediated increase in Treg frequency. Unlike immature T cells, Tregs are resistant to GC-induced cell death in vivo and account for a greater proportion of T cells in mice treated with GC [23]. Moreover, expansion of tTregs by IL-10 upregulation and the facilitated generation of peripheral Tregs (pTregs) have been observed [12, 25, 75]. To this end, GCs synergize with transforming growth factor-β signaling in FoxP3 induction through induction of GILZ and consequent SMAD2 phosphorylation, which is necessary for the GC-induced increase in Treg number [15, 47, 75].

Effects on Effector T Cells

GCs affect peripheral immune responses by inhibiting or modulating effector T cell activation at several stages of the activation cascade (section "Molecular mechanisms of glucocorticoids"). Specifically, reports have described GC-mediated transcriptional regulation of TCR complex proteins [59, 64, 82] as well as modulation of TCR function and signal transduction [9, 26, 53, 65]. In particular, GCs modulate kinase expression and activity [73, 99]. Because the peripheral responsiveness of T cells appears to be regulated by the quantity and quality of intracellular signals triggered by TCR activation, the interference of GCs on TCR signaling contributes to their effect on T cells.

Another interesting GC-mediated effect is a shift in the balance of the immune response from a Th1 to a Th2 type [78]. In the initial stages of an immune response, naive cells that are committed to activation and differentiation into either Th1 or Th2 phenotypes are initially suppressed in the presence of GCs, which is consistent with their general immunosuppressive action. Indeed, GCs inhibit both T-bet, which is selectively expressed in Th1 cells, by transrepression, and GATA3, which is selectively expressed in Th2 cells, by inhibiting p38 MAPK phosphorylation. However, the greater sensitivity of T-bet to GC inhibition favors Th2 development, particularly during long-term GC treatment [49]. The GC-dependent upregulation of Itk, a Tec kinase favoring Th2 polarization, may be another polarization mechanism of GC [73].

GCs affect both Th17 polarization and function by modulating cytokines such as IL-23, IL-6, and IL-17 [39, 62]. It was also recently demonstrated that the aberrant Th17/Th1 balance in patients with SLE is linked to GC use [74]. Investigations using specific conditional knockout models will likely identify a clear correlation between Th17 and GC action.

A third GC-mediated effect on mature T cells is apoptotic cell death. The degree of activation and the timing of GC exposure (before, during, or after activation) render T cells sensitive or resistant to GC-induced apoptosis [105].

Effects on Thymocytes

GC actions in thymocytes have been the subject of several studies. However, several controversies remain. It has long been known that high systemic GC levels lead to thymus involution whereas low concentrations result in oversized thymus. During development, immature double-negative thymocytes ($CD4^{-}CD8^{-}$) progress to the double-positive phenotype ($CD4^{+}CD8^{+}$) and undergo positive or negative selection depending on mild or strong binding, respectively, between their major histocompatibility complexes and self-antigens. At this stage, double-positive thymocytes are highly sensitive to GC-induced apoptosis that, in turn, can be antagonized by TCR signaling and vice versa (termed mutual antagonism) [4]. A number of genetically modified mouse models with altered GRs have been produced to help understand the role of GCs in thymocyte death by neglect. These studies have yielded conflicting results. It seems reasonable to conclude that GR triggering is dispensable for thymocyte development under physiological conditions but may affect thymocyte turnover under stress conditions, such as infection, or during prolonged GC treatment [77, 102]. This topic has been previously discussed in depth [81].

Effects on the Cells of Innate Immunity

Adaptive immunity is not the only player in autoimmunity. In fact, innate immune system cells, including dendritic cells (DCs), natural killer (NK) cells, NK T lymphocytes, and macrophages, also modulate self-tolerance. Epithelial and endothelial cells have also been implicated in the pathogenesis of autoimmune diseases. GCs are able to influence the function of these cells and were recently found to affect TLR signaling [68], thus contributing to the counteraction of autoimmune diseases.

GC-treated immature DCs are unable to undergo full maturation and prime Th1 cells efficiently [56]. After GC exposure, mature DCs show a decreased ability to present antigens and activate T cells and are reprogrammed into the so-called tolerogenic DC. At the molecular level, such an orientation to tolerance is driven, at least in part, by GILZ upregulation, which can prevent the expression of CD80, CD86, and CD83 as well as DC production of inflammatory chemokines. This interferes with the NF-κB pathway, which allows for DC maturation, and simultaneously induces IL-10 production [41, 80]. GC-treated DCs also possess the capacity to convert CD4 T cells into IL-10-secreting Tregs, potently suppressing the proliferation of responder T cells [97].

During inflammatory processes, macrophages resolve inflammation in several ways, including recognition and phagocytosis of apoptotic cells (such as dead neutrophils). Endogenous GCs can exert distinct effects on macrophages depending on their concentration and the functional status of the macrophages. Some studies suggest that GCs reduce rolling, adhesion, and transmigration of proinflammatory monocytes by lowering the expression of adhesion molecules such as β2 integrins [lymphocyte function-associated antigen-1 (LFA-1) and macrophage-1 antigen (Mac-1)] and selectins, which interact with their endothelial counterparts on endothelial cells [51]. Other studies suggest that GC treatment promotes migration of anti-inflammatory monocytes, inducing their differentiation toward specific subtypes with particular anti-inflammatory phenotypes [37]. Moreover, GCs exert immunostimulatory effects on macrophages favoring cell uptake [51, 106]. Interestingly, this occurs even in alveolar macrophages, in which cell uptake is inhibited by the lung environment [57].

Acute cortisol that is released following stress or intravenous GC injection causes a profound depletion of eosinophils and basophils due to apoptosis, thus preventing tissue invasion. By contrast, systemic GCs elicit opposing effects on neutrophils by increasing the number of peripheral neutrophils, as well as their bone marrow progenitors [96], and delaying spontaneous apoptosis. Notably, GCs reduce reactive oxygen species generation and proinflammatory cytokine expression in peripheral neutrophils [43].

Stress decreases NK cell activity, and recently the molecular mechanisms of GR-mediated gene suppression have begun to be unraveled in these cells [20]. However, a recent report describes a synergistic effect of GCs with IL-15 in increasing the proliferation of human peripheral blood NK cells and protecting against cytokine-induced cell death. This is an emerging topic because of the potential use of NK cells as a powerful tool in cancer immunotherapy [63].

Conclusions

GC-induced immunomodulation has emerged as a multistep mechanism that acts on several components of the immune system, negatively affecting both innate and adaptive responses. However, in some contexts, GCs may have immunomodulatory rather than immunosuppressive effects. Future research will aim at clarifying the pathophysiology of autoimmune diseases, and new drugs that share the benefits of GCs without the adverse side effects should improve pharmacological treatment. In the interim, efforts should be made to improve treatment protocols, which may enhance the therapeutic outcomes of available GCs.

References

1. Alunno A, Bartoloni E, Bistoni O, Nocentini G, Ronchetti S, Caterbi S, Valentini V, Riccardi C, Gerli R (2012) Balance between regulatory T and Th17 cells in systemic lupus erythematosus: the old and the new. Clin Dev Immunol 2012:823085. doi:10.1155/2012/823085
2. Alunno A, Petrillo MG, Nocentini G, Bistoni O, Bartoloni E, Caterbi S, Bianchini R, Baldini C, Nicoletti I, Riccardi C, Gerli R (2013) Characterization of a new regulatory CD4+ T cell subset in primary Sjogren's syndrome. Rheumatology (Oxford) 52(8):1387–1396. doi:10.1093/rheumatology/ket179

3. Aristimuno C, Navarro J, de Andres C, Martinez-Gines L, Gimenez-Roldan S, Fernandez-Cruz E, Sanchez-Ramon S (2008) Expansion of regulatory CD8+ T-lymphocytes and fall of activated CD8+ T-lymphocytes after i.v. methyl-prednisolone for multiple sclerosis relapse. J Neuroimmunol 204(1–2):131–135. doi:10.1016/j.jneuroim.2008.08.009
4. Ashwell JD, Lu FW, Vacchio MS (2000) Glucocorticoids in T cell development and function*. Annu Rev Immunol 18:309–345. doi:10.1146/annurev.immunol.18.1.309
5. Auphan N, DiDonato JA, Rosette C, Helmberg A, Karin M (1995) Immunosuppression by glucocorticoids: inhibition of NF-kappa B activity through induction of I kappa B synthesis. Science 270(5234):286–290
6. Ayroldi E, Cannarile L, Migliorati G, Nocentini G, Delfino DV, Riccardi C (2012) Mechanisms of the anti-inflammatory effects of glucocorticoids: genomic and nongenomic interference with MAPK signaling pathways. FASEB J 26(12):4805–4820. doi:10.1096/fj.12-216382
7. Ayroldi E, Migliorati G, Bruscoli S, Marchetti C, Zollo O, Cannarile L, D'Adamio F, Riccardi C (2001) Modulation of T-cell activation by the glucocorticoid-induced leucine zipper factor via inhibition of nuclear factor kappaB. Blood 98(3):743–753
8. Ayroldi E, Riccardi C (2009) Glucocorticoid-induced leucine zipper (GILZ): a new important mediator of glucocorticoid action. FASEB J 23(11):3649–3658. doi:10.1096/fj.09-134684
9. Ayroldi E, Zollo O, Bastianelli A, Marchetti C, Agostini M, Di Virgilio R, Riccardi C (2007) GILZ mediates the antiproliferative activity of glucocorticoids by negative regulation of Ras signaling. J Clin Invest 117(6):1605–1615. doi:10.1172/JCI30724
10. Ayroldi E, Zollo O, Macchiarulo A, Di Marco B, Marchetti C, Riccardi C (2002) Glucocorticoid-induced leucine zipper inhibits the Raf-extracellular signal-regulated kinase pathway by binding to Raf-1. Mol Cell Biol 22(22):7929–7941
11. Azab NA, Bassyouni IH, Emad Y, Abd El-Wahab GA, Hamdy G, Mashahit MA (2008) CD4+CD25+ regulatory T cells (TREG) in systemic lupus erythematosus (SLE) patients: the possible influence of treatment with corticosteroids. Clin Immunol 127(2):151–157. doi:10.1016/j.clim.2007.12.010
12. Barrat FJ, Cua DJ, Boonstra A, Richards DF, Crain C, Savelkoul HF, de Waal-Malefyt R, Coffman RL, Hawrylowicz CM, O'Garra A (2002) In vitro generation of interleukin 10-producing regulatory CD4(+) T cells is induced by immunosuppressive drugs and inhibited by T helper type 1 (Th1)- and Th2-inducing cytokines. J Exp Med 195(5): 603–616
13. Baumann S, Dostert A, Novac N, Bauer A, Schmid W, Fas SC, Krueger A, Heinzel T, Kirchhoff S, Schutz G, Krammer PH (2005) Glucocorticoids inhibit activation-induced cell death (AICD) via direct DNA-dependent repression of the CD95 ligand gene by a glucocorticoid receptor dimer. Blood 106(2):617–625. doi:10.1182/blood-2004-11-4390
14. Beck IM, Vanden Berghe W, Vermeulen L, Yamamoto KR, Haegeman G, De Bosscher K (2009) Crosstalk in inflammation: the interplay of glucocorticoid receptor-based mechanisms and kinases and phosphatases. Endocr Rev 30(7):830–882. doi:10.1210/er.2009-0013
15. Bereshchenko O, Coppo M, Bruscoli S, Biagioli M, Cimino M, Frammartino T, Sorcini D, Venanzi A, Di Sante M, Riccardi C (2014) GILZ promotes production of peripherally induced treg cells and mediates the crosstalk between glucocorticoids and TGF-beta signaling. Cell Rep 7(2):464–475. doi:10.1016/j.celrep.2014.03.004
16. Bianchini R, Nocentini G, Krausz LT, Fettucciari K, Coaccioli S, Ronchetti S, Riccardi C (2006) Modulation of pro- and antiapoptotic molecules in double-positive (CD4+CD8+) thymocytes following dexamethasone treatment. J Pharmacol Exp Ther 319(2):887–897. doi:10.1124/jpet.106.108480
17. Biddie SC, Conway-Campbell BL, Lightman SL (2012) Dynamic regulation of glucocorticoid signalling in health and disease. Rheumatology (Oxford) 51(3):403–412. doi:10.1093/rheumatology/ker215
18. Bolon B (2012) Cellular and molecular mechanisms of autoimmune disease. Toxicol Pathol 40(2):216–229. doi:10.1177/0192623311428481
19. Braitch M, Harikrishnan S, Robins RA, Nichols C, Fahey AJ, Showe L, Constantinescu CS (2009) Glucocorticoids increase CD4CD25 cell percentage and Foxp3 expression

in patients with multiple sclerosis. Acta Neurol Scand 119(4):239–245. doi:10.1111/j.1600-0404.2008.01090.x
20. Bush KA, Krukowski K, Eddy JL, Janusek LW, Mathews HL (2012) Glucocorticoid receptor mediated suppression of natural killer cell activity: identification of associated deacetylase and corepressor molecules. Cell Immunol 275(1–2):80–89. doi:10.1016/j.cellimm.2012.02.014
21. Busillo JM, Cidlowski JA (2013) The five Rs of glucocorticoid action during inflammation: ready, reinforce, repress, resolve, and restore. Trends Endocrinol Metab 24(3):109–119. doi:10.1016/j.tem.2012.11.005
22. Chauhan S, Leach CH, Kunz S, Bloom JW, Miesfeld RL (2003) Glucocorticoid regulation of human eosinophil gene expression. J Steroid Biochem Mol Biol 84(4):441–452
23. Chen X, Murakami T, Oppenheim JJ, Howard OM (2004) Differential response of murine CD4+CD25+ and CD4+CD25- T cells to dexamethasone-induced cell death. Eur J Immunol 34(3):859–869
24. Chen X, Oppenheim JJ, Winkler-Pickett RT, Ortaldo JR, Howard OM (2006) Glucocorticoid amplifies IL-2-dependent expansion of functional FoxP3(+)CD4(+)CD25(+) T regulatory cells in vivo and enhances their capacity to suppress EAE. Eur J Immunol 36(8):2139–2149. doi:10.1002/eji.200635873
25. Chung IY, Dong HF, Zhang X, Hassanein NM, Howard OM, Oppenheim JJ, Chen X (2004) Effects of IL-7 and dexamethasone: induction of CD25, the high affinity IL-2 receptor, on human CD4+ cells. Cell Immunol 232(1–2):57–63. doi:10.1016/j.cellimm.2005.01.011
26. Cifone MG, Migliorati G, Parroni R, Marchetti C, Millimaggi D, Santoni A, Riccardi C (1999) Dexamethasone-induced thymocyte apoptosis: apoptotic signal involves the sequential activation of phosphoinositide-specific phospholipase C, acidic sphingomyelinase, and caspases. Blood 93(7):2282–2296
27. Croxtall JD, Choudhury Q, Flower RJ (2000) Glucocorticoids act within minutes to inhibit recruitment of signalling factors to activated EGF receptors through a receptor-dependent, transcription-independent mechanism. Br J Pharmacol 130(2):289–298. doi:10.1038/sj.bjp.0703272
28. D'Adamio F, Zollo O, Moraca R, Ayroldi E, Bruscoli S, Bartoli A, Cannarile L, Migliorati G, Riccardi C (1997) A new dexamethasone-induced gene of the leucine zipper family protects T lymphocytes from TCR/CD3-activated cell death. Immunity 7(6):803–812
29. Damsker JM, Hansen AM, Caspi RR (2010) Th1 and Th17 cells: adversaries and collaborators. Ann N Y Acad Sci 1183:211–221. doi:10.1111/j.1749-6632.2009.05133.x
30. Das H, Kumar A, Lin Z, Patino WD, Hwang PM, Feinberg MW, Majumder PK, Jain MK (2006) Kruppel-like factor 2 (KLF2) regulates proinflammatory activation of monocytes. Proc Natl Acad Sci U S A 103(17):6653–6658. doi:10.1073/pnas.0508235103
31. De Bosscher K, Vanden Berghe W, Haegeman G (2000) Mechanisms of anti-inflammatory action and of immunosuppression by glucocorticoids: negative interference of activated glucocorticoid receptor with transcription factors. J Neuroimmunol 109(1):16–22
32. De Bosscher K, Vanden Berghe W, Haegeman G (2006) Cross-talk between nuclear receptors and nuclear factor kappaB. Oncogene 25(51):6868–6886. doi:10.1038/sj.onc.1209935
33. de Paz B, Prado C, Alperi-Lopez M, Ballina-Garcia FJ, Rodriguez-Carrio J, Lopez P, Suarez A (2012) Effects of glucocorticoid treatment on CD25(−)FOXP3(+) population and cytokine-producing cells in rheumatoid arthritis. Rheumatology (Oxford) 51(7):1198–1207. doi:10.1093/rheumatology/kes039
34. Delfino DV, Agostini M, Spinicelli S, Vacca C, Riccardi C (2006) Inhibited cell death, NF-kappaB activity and increased IL-10 in TCR-triggered thymocytes of transgenic mice overexpressing the glucocorticoid-induced protein GILZ. Int Immunopharmacol 6(7):1126–1134. doi:10.1016/j.intimp.2006.02.001
35. Di Marco B, Massetti M, Bruscoli S, Macchiarulo A, Di Virgilio R, Velardi E, Donato V, Migliorati G, Riccardi C (2007) Glucocorticoid-induced leucine zipper (GILZ)/NF-kappaB interaction: role of GILZ homo-dimerization and C-terminal domain. Nucleic Acids Res 35(2):517–528

36. Dostert A, Heinzel T (2004) Negative glucocorticoid receptor response elements and their role in glucocorticoid action. Curr Pharm Des 10(23):2807–2816
37. Ehrchen J, Steinmuller L, Barczyk K, Tenbrock K, Nacken W, Eisenacher M, Nordhues U, Sorg C, Sunderkotter C, Roth J (2007) Glucocorticoids induce differentiation of a specifically activated, anti-inflammatory subtype of human monocytes. Blood 109(3):1265–1274. doi:10.1182/blood-2006-02-001115
38. Ferlazzo V, D'Agostino P, Milano S, Caruso R, Feo S, Cillari E, Parente L (2003) Anti-inflammatory effects of annexin-1: stimulation of IL-10 release and inhibition of nitric oxide synthesis. Int Immunopharmacol 3(10–11):1363–1369. doi:10.1016/S1567-5769(03)00133-4
39. Flammer JR, Rogatsky I (2011) Minireview: glucocorticoids in autoimmunity: unexpected targets and mechanisms. Mol Endocrinol 25(7):1075–1086. doi:10.1210/me.2011-0068
40. Gerli R, Nocentini G, Alunno A, Bocci EB, Bianchini R, Bistoni O, Riccardi C (2009) Identification of regulatory T cells in systemic lupus erythematosus. Autoimmun Rev 8(5):426–430. doi:10.1016/j.autrev.2009.01.004
41. Hamdi H, Godot V, Maillot MC, Prejean MV, Cohen N, Krzysiek R, Lemoine FM, Zou W, Emilie D (2007) Induction of antigen-specific regulatory T lymphocytes by human dendritic cells expressing the glucocorticoid-induced leucine zipper. Blood 110(1):211–219. doi:10.1182/blood-2006-10-052506
42. Haribhai D, Williams JB, Jia S, Nickerson D, Schmitt EG, Edwards B, Ziegelbauer J, Yassai M, Li SH, Relland LM, Wise PM, Chen A, Zheng YQ, Simpson PM, Gorski J, Salzman NH, Hessner MJ, Chatila TA, Williams CB (2011) A requisite role for induced regulatory T cells in tolerance based on expanding antigen receptor diversity. Immunity 35(1):109–122. doi:10.1016/j.immuni.2011.03.029
43. Hirsch G, Lavoie-Lamoureux A, Beauchamp G, Lavoie JP (2012) Neutrophils are not less sensitive than other blood leukocytes to the genomic effects of glucocorticoids. PLoS One 7(9):e44606. doi:10.1371/journal.pone.0044606
44. Hu Y, Tian W, Zhang LL, Liu H, Yin GP, He BS, Mao XM (2012) Function of regulatory T-cells improved by dexamethasone in Graves' disease. Eur J Endocrinol 166(4):641–646. doi:10.1530/EJE-11-0879
45. Jing Y, Hou Y, Song Y, Yin J (2012) Methylprednisolone improves the survival of new neurons following transient cerebral ischemia in rats. Acta Neurobiol Exp 72(3):240–252
46. John S, Sabo PJ, Thurman RE, Sung MH, Biddie SC, Johnson TA, Hager GL, Stamatoyannopoulos JA (2011) Chromatin accessibility pre-determines glucocorticoid receptor binding patterns. Nat Genet 43(3):264–268. doi:10.1038/ng.759
47. Karagiannidis C, Akdis M, Holopainen P, Woolley NJ, Hense G, Ruckert B, Mantel PY, Menz G, Akdis CA, Blaser K, Schmidt-Weber CB (2004) Glucocorticoids upregulate FOXP3 expression and regulatory T cells in asthma. J Allergy Clin Immunol 114(6):1425–1433. doi:10.1016/j.jaci.2004.07.014
48. Lawson CA, Brown AK, Bejarano V, Douglas SH, Burgoyne CH, Greenstein AS, Boylston AW, Emery P, Ponchel F, Isaacs JD (2006) Early rheumatoid arthritis is associated with a deficit in the CD4+CD25high regulatory T cell population in peripheral blood. Rheumatology (Oxford) 45(10):1210–1217. doi:10.1093/rheumatology/kel089
49. Liberman AC, Druker J, Refojo D, Holsboer F, Arzt E (2009) Glucocorticoids inhibit GATA-3 phosphorylation and activity in T cells. FASEB J 23(5):1558–1571. doi:10.1096/fj.08-121236
50. Liberman AC, Refojo D, Druker J, Toscano M, Rein T, Holsboer F, Arzt E (2007) The activated glucocorticoid receptor inhibits the transcription factor T-bet by direct protein-protein interaction. FASEB J 21(4):1177–1188. doi:10.1096/fj.06-7452com
51. Lim HY, Muller N, Herold MJ, van den Brandt J, Reichardt HM (2007) Glucocorticoids exert opposing effects on macrophage function dependent on their concentration. Immunology 122(1):47–53. doi:10.1111/j.1365-2567.2007.02611.x
52. Lowenberg M, Verhaar AP, Bilderbeek J, Marle J, Buttgereit F, Peppelenbosch MP, van Deventer SJ, Hommes DW (2006) Glucocorticoids cause rapid dissociation of a T-cell-

receptor-associated protein complex containing LCK and FYN. EMBO Rep 7(10):1023–1029. doi:10.1038/sj.embor.7400775
53. Lowenberg M, Verhaar AP, van den Brink GR, Hommes DW (2007) Glucocorticoid signaling: a nongenomic mechanism for T-cell immunosuppression. Trends Mol Med 13(4):158–163. doi:10.1016/j.molmed.2007.02.001
54. Mann CL, Cidlowski JA (2001) Glucocorticoids regulate plasma membrane potential during rat thymocyte apoptosis in vivo and in vitro. Endocrinology 142(1):421–429. doi:10.1210/endo.142.1.7904
55. Marchetti MC, Di Marco B, Cifone G, Migliorati G, Riccardi C (2003) Dexamethasone-induced apoptosis of thymocytes: role of glucocorticoid receptor-associated Src kinase and caspase-8 activation. Blood 101(2):585–593. doi:10.1182/blood-2002-06-1779
56. Matyszak MK, Citterio S, Rescigno M, Ricciardi-Castagnoli P (2000) Differential effects of corticosteroids during different stages of dendritic cell maturation. Eur J Immunol 30(4):1233–1242. doi:10.1002/(SICI)1521-4141(200004)30:4<1233::AID-IMMU1233>3.0.CO;2-F
57. McCubbrey AL, Sonstein J, Ames TM, Freeman CM, Curtis JL (2012) Glucocorticoids relieve collectin-driven suppression of apoptotic cell uptake in murine alveolar macrophages through downregulation of SIRPalpha. J Immunol 189(1):112–119. doi:10.4049/jimmunol.1200984
58. McKay LI, Cidlowski JA (1998) Cross-talk between nuclear factor-kappa B and the steroid hormone receptors: mechanisms of mutual antagonism. Mol Endocrinol 12(1):45–56
59. Migliorati G, Bartoli A, Nocentini G, Ronchetti S, Moraca R, Riccardi C (1997) Effect of dexamethasone on T-cell receptor/CD3 expression. Mol Cell Biochem 167(1–2):135–144
60. Miner JN, Yamamoto KR (1991) Regulatory crosstalk at composite response elements. Trends Biochem Sci 16(11):423–426
61. Mittelstadt PR, Ashwell JD (2001) Inhibition of AP-1 by the glucocorticoid-inducible protein GILZ. J Biol Chem 276(31):29603–29610. doi:10.1074/jbc.M101522200
62. Momcilovic M, Miljkovic Z, Popadic D, Markovic M, Savic E, Ramic Z, Miljkovic D, Mostarica-Stojkovic M (2008) Methylprednisolone inhibits interleukin-17 and interferon-gamma expression by both naive and primed T cells. BMC Immunol 9:47. doi:10.1186/1471-2172-9-47
63. Moustaki A, Argyropoulos KV, Baxevanis CN, Papamichail M, Perez SA (2011) Effect of the simultaneous administration of glucocorticoids and IL-15 on human NK cell phenotype, proliferation and function. Cancer Immunol Immunother 60(12):1683–1695. doi:10.1007/s00262-011-1067-6
64. Nambiar MP, Enyedy EJ, Fisher CU, Warke VG, Juang YT, Tsokos GC (2001) Dexamethasone modulates TCR zeta chain expression and antigen receptor-mediated early signaling events in human T lymphocytes. Cell Immunol 208(1):62–71. doi:10.1006/cimm.2001.1761
65. Nambiar MP, Enyedy EJ, Fisher CU, Warke VG, Tsokos GC (2001) High dose of dexamethasone upregulates TCR/CD3-induced calcium response independent of TCR zeta chain expression in human T lymphocytes. J Cell Biochem 83(3):401–413
66. Nocentini G, Alunno A, Petrillo MG, Bistoni O, Bartoloni E, Caterbi S, Ronchetti S, Migliorati G, Riccardi C, Gerli R (2014) Expansion of regulatory GITR+CD25 low/-CD4+ T cells in systemic lupus erythematosus patients. Arthritis Res Ther 16(5):444.
67. Novac N, Baus D, Dostert A, Heinzel T (2006) Competition between glucocorticoid receptor and NFkappaB for control of the human FasL promoter. FASEB J 20(8):1074–1081. doi:10.1096/fj.05-5457com
68. O'Neill LA (2008) When signaling pathways collide: positive and negative regulation of toll-like receptor signal transduction. Immunity 29(1):12–20. doi:10.1016/j.immuni.2008.06.004
69. Oakley RH, Jewell CM, Yudt MR, Bofetiado DM, Cidlowski JA (1999) The dominant negative activity of the human glucocorticoid receptor beta isoform. Specificity and mechanisms of action. J Biol Chem 274(39):27857–27866
70. Oppong E, Hedde PN, Sekula-Neuner S, Yang L, Brinkmann F, Dorlich RM, Hirtz M, Fuchs H, Nienhaus GU, Cato AC (2014) Localization and dynamics of glucocorticoid receptor at

the plasma membrane of activated mast cells. Small 10(10):1991–1998. doi:10.1002/smll.201303677

71. Palinkas L, Talaber G, Boldizsar F, Bartis D, Nemeth P, Berki T (2008) Developmental shift in TcR-mediated rescue of thymocytes from glucocorticoid-induced apoptosis. Immunobiology 213(1):39–50. doi:10.1016/j.imbio.2007.06.004
72. Pecci A, Scholz A, Pelster D, Beato M (1997) Progestins prevent apoptosis in a rat endometrial cell line and increase the ratio of bcl-XL to bcl-XS. J Biol Chem 272(18):11791–11798
73. Petrillo MG, Fettucciari K, Montuschi P, Ronchetti S, Cari L, Migliorati G, Mazzon E, Bereshchenko O, Bruscoli S, Nocentini G, Riccardi C (2014) Transcriptional regulation of kinases downstream of the T cell receptor: another immunomodulatory mechanism of glucocorticoids. BMC Pharmacol Toxicol 15:35. doi:10.1186/2050-6511-15-35
74. Prado C, de Paz B, Gomez J, Lopez P, Rodriguez-Carrio J, Suarez A (2011) Glucocorticoids enhance Th17/Th1 imbalance and signal transducer and activator of transcription 3 expression in systemic lupus erythematosus patients. Rheumatology (Oxford) 50(10):1794–1801. doi:10.1093/rheumatology/ker227
75. Prado C, Gomez J, Lopez P, de Paz B, Gutierrez C, Suarez A (2011) Dexamethasone upregulates FOXP3 expression without increasing regulatory activity. Immunobiology 216(3):386–392. doi:10.1016/j.imbio.2010.06.013
76. Pratt WB, Toft DO (1997) Steroid receptor interactions with heat shock protein and immunophilin chaperones. Endocr Rev 18(3):306–360
77. Purton JF, Boyd RL, Cole TJ, Godfrey DI (2000) Intrathymic T cell development and selection proceeds normally in the absence of glucocorticoid receptor signaling. Immunity 13(2):179–186
78. Ramirez F, Fowell DJ, Puklavec M, Simmonds S, Mason D (1996) Glucocorticoids promote a TH2 cytokine response by CD4+ T cells in vitro. J Immunol 156(7):2406–2412
79. Revollo JR, Cidlowski JA (2009) Mechanisms generating diversity in glucocorticoid receptor signaling. Ann N Y Acad Sci 1179:167–178. doi:10.1111/j.1749-6632.2009.04986.x
80. Riccardi C, Bruscoli S, Ayroldi E, Agostini M, Migliorati G (2001) GILZ, a glucocorticoid hormone induced gene, modulates T lymphocytes activation and death through interaction with NF-kB. Adv Exp Med Biol 495:31–39
81. Ronchetti S, Migliorati G, Riccardi C (2014) Glucocorticoid-Induced Immunomodulation. In: E. Corsini and H. van Loveren (eds.) Mol Immunotoxicol. Wiley Blackwell, p.209–226 doi:10.1002/9783527676965.ch10
82. Ronchetti S, Nocentini G, Giunchi L, Bartoli A, Moraca R, Riccardi C, Migliorati G (1997) Short-term dexamethasone treatment modulates the expression of the murine TCR zeta gene locus. Cell Immunol 178(2):124–131. doi:10.1006/cimm.1997.1131
83. Schmidt S, Rainer J, Ploner C, Presul E, Riml S, Kofler R (2004) Glucocorticoid-induced apoptosis and glucocorticoid resistance: molecular mechanisms and clinical relevance. Cell Death Differ 11(Suppl 1):S45–S55. doi:10.1038/sj.cdd.4401456
84. Shipp LE, Lee JV, Yu CY, Pufall M, Zhang P, Scott DK, Wang JC (2010) Transcriptional regulation of human dual specificity protein phosphatase 1 (DUSP1) gene by glucocorticoids. PLoS One 5(10):e13754. doi:10.1371/journal.pone.0013754
85. Sionov RV, Cohen O, Kfir S, Zilberman Y, Yefenof E (2006) Role of mitochondrial glucocorticoid receptor in glucocorticoid-induced apoptosis. J Exp Med 203(1):189–201. doi:10.1084/jem.20050433
86. Smoak K, Cidlowski JA (2006) Glucocorticoids regulate tristetraprolin synthesis and post-transcriptionally regulate tumor necrosis factor alpha inflammatory signaling. Mol Cell Biol 26(23):9126–9135. doi:10.1128/MCB. 00679-06
87. Souza DG, Fagundes CT, Amaral FA, Cisalpino D, Sousa LP, Vieira AT, Pinho V, Nicoli JR, Vieira LQ, Fierro IM, Teixeira MM (2007) The required role of endogenously produced lipoxin A4 and annexin-1 for the production of IL-10 and inflammatory hyporesponsiveness in mice. J Immunol 179(12):8533–8543
88. Stell BM, Brickley SG, Tang CY, Farrant M, Mody I (2003) Neuroactive steroids reduce neuronal excitability by selectively enhancing tonic inhibition mediated by delta subunit-

containing GABAA receptors. Proc Natl Acad Sci U S A 100(24):14439–14444. doi:10.1073/pnas.2435457100
89. Stocklin E, Wissler M, Gouilleux F, Groner B (1996) Functional interactions between Stat5 and the glucocorticoid receptor. Nature 383(6602):726–728. doi:10.1038/383726a0
90. Strehl C, Buttgereit F (2014) Unraveling the functions of the membrane-bound glucocorticoid receptors: first clues on origin and functional activity. Ann N Y Acad Sci 1318(1):1–6. doi:10.1111/nyas.12364
91. Suarez A, Lopez P, Gomez J, Gutierrez C (2006) Enrichment of CD4+ CD25high T cell population in patients with systemic lupus erythematosus treated with glucocorticoids. Ann Rheum Dis 65(11):1512–1517. doi:10.1136/ard.2005.049924
92. Surjit M, Ganti KP, Mukherji A, Ye T, Hua G, Metzger D, Li M, Chambon P (2011) Widespread negative response elements mediate direct repression by agonist-liganded glucocorticoid receptor. Cell 145(2):224–241. doi:10.1016/j.cell.2011.03.027
93. Tasker JG, Di S, Malcher-Lopes R (2006) Minireview: rapid glucocorticoid signaling via membrane-associated receptors. Endocrinology 147(12):5549–5556. doi:10.1210/en.2006-0981
94. Thompson JA, Perry D, Brusko TM (2012) Autologous regulatory T cells for the treatment of type 1 diabetes. Curr Diab Rep 12(5):623–632. doi:10.1007/s11892-012-0304-5
95. Treccani G, Musazzi L, Perego C, Milanese M, Nava N, Bonifacino T, Lamanna J, Malgaroli A, Drago F, Racagni G, Nyengaard JR, Wegener G, Bonanno G, Popoli M (2014) Stress and corticosterone increase the readily releasable pool of glutamate vesicles in synaptic terminals of prefrontal and frontal cortex. Mol Psychiatry 19(4):433–443. doi:10.1038/mp.2014.5
96. Trottier MD, Newsted MM, King LE, Fraker PJ (2008) Natural glucocorticoids induce expansion of all developmental stages of murine bone marrow granulocytes without inhibiting function. Proc Natl Acad Sci U S A 105(6):2028–2033. doi:10.1073/pnas.0712003105
97. Unger WW, Laban S, Kleijwegt FS, van der Slik AR, Roep BO (2009) Induction of Treg by monocyte-derived DC modulated by vitamin D3 or dexamethasone: differential role for PD-L1. Eur J Immunol 39(11):3147–3159. doi:10.1002/eji.200839103
98. van Batenburg MF, Li H, Polman JA, Lachize S, Datson NA, Bussemaker HJ, Meijer OC (2010) Paired hormone response elements predict caveolin-1 as a glucocorticoid target gene. PLoS One 5(1):e8839. doi:10.1371/journal.pone.0008839
99. Van Laethem F, Baus E, Smyth LA, Andris F, Bex F, Urbain J, Kioussis D, Leo O (2001) Glucocorticoids attenuate T cell receptor signaling. J Exp Med 193(7):803–814
100. Vandevyver S, Dejager L, Libert C (2012) On the trail of the glucocorticoid receptor: into the nucleus and back. Traffic 13(3):364–374. doi:10.1111/j.1600-0854.2011.01288.x
101. Vandevyver S, Dejager L, Tuckermann J, Libert C (2013) New insights into the anti-inflammatory mechanisms of glucocorticoids: an emerging role for glucocorticoid-receptor-mediated transactivation. Endocrinology 154(3):993–1007. doi:10.1210/en.2012-2045
102. Wiegers GJ, Kaufmann M, Tischner D, Villunger A (2011) Shaping the T-cell repertoire: a matter of life and death. Immunol Cell Biol 89(1):33–39. doi:10.1038/icb.2010.127
103. Wu I, Shin SC, Cao Y, Bender IK, Jafari N, Feng G, Lin S, Cidlowski JA, Schleimer RP, Lu NZ (2013) Selective glucocorticoid receptor translational isoforms reveal glucocorticoid-induced apoptotic transcriptomes. Cell Death Dis 4:e453. doi:10.1038/cddis.2012.193
104. Yang N, Zhang W, Shi XM (2008) Glucocorticoid-induced leucine zipper (GILZ) mediates glucocorticoid action and inhibits inflammatory cytokine-induced COX-2 expression. J Cell Biochem 103(6):1760–1771. doi:10.1002/jcb.21562
105. Zacharchuk CM, Mercep M, Chakraborti PK, Simons SS Jr, Ashwell JD (1990) Programmed T lymphocyte death. Cell activation- and steroid-induced pathways are mutually antagonistic. J Immunol 145(12):4037–4045
106. Zhou JY, Zhong HJ, Yang C, Yan J, Wang HY, Jiang JX (2010) Corticosterone exerts immunostimulatory effects on macrophages via endoplasmic reticulum stress. Br J Surg 97(2):281–293. doi:10.1002/bjs.6820

The Clinical Pharmacology of Past, Present, and Future Glucocorticoids

Giuseppe Nocentini, Simona Ronchetti, Stefano Bruscoli, and Carlo Riccardi

Introduction

Glucocorticoids (GCs) inhibit early and late manifestations of acute inflammation and modulate subsequent repair by acting on a variety of immune and nonimmune cell functions, including extravasation and migration. Moreover, GCs are immunosuppressive agents. Therefore, GCs are widely used to treat inflammatory conditions, allergies, and autoimmune diseases and to prevent or treat acute and chronic transplant rejection and graft-versus-host disease. The proapoptotic effects of GCs on immune cells are useful in the treatment of hematological malignancies.

At clinical doses, all effects of GCs result from the interaction of GCs with their receptor (GR), which is expressed in nearly all cell types. The GR is located in the cytoplasm, where it is found in a multimeric chaperone complex or bound to transmembrane receptors, kinases, or other cellular structures. Upon GR activation by GCs, several pathways are activated that promote genomic and nongenomic effects. Genomic effects require several minutes to occur, and they fully impact cell function after several hours or days. However, nongenomic effects have a very rapid manifestation. Genomic effects include increased transcription of some genes and decreased transcription of others. Increased gene transcription is primarily caused by homodimerization of an activated GR and its binding to short sequences of DNA called glucocorticoid-responsive elements (GREs), whereas decreased gene transcription predominantly results from etherodimerization of activated GRs with transcription factors, thus inhibiting gene transcription promoted by these transcription factors. Another relevant mechanism by which GCs downregulate gene transcription is by upregulating the inhibitors of transcription factors and the interaction with

G. Nocentini • S. Ronchetti • S. Bruscoli • C. Riccardi (✉)
Section of Pharmacology, Department of Medicine, University of Perugia, Building D, 2nd Floor, Severi Square 1, San Sisto, Perugia I-06132, Italy
e-mail: giuseppe.nocentini@unipg.it; carlo.riccardi@unipg.it

R. Cimaz (ed.), *Systemic Corticosteroids for Inflammatory Disorders in Pediatrics*, DOI 10.1007/978-3-319-16056-6_5

negative GREs. A detailed overview of the genomic and nongenomic effects of GCs is presented in another chapter of this book and elsewhere [2, 5, 13, 61, 70, 71, 74].

GCs have powerful anti-inflammatory effects because they inhibit the production of proinflammatory factors, including cytokines, chemokines, nitric oxide, and prostaglandins, and modulate endothelial function [18, 42, 74]. This affects virtually all cells of the adaptive and innate immune system. GC treatment has several effects on T-cell subsets. In a clinical setting, the effects on regulatory T cells and T helper cell polarization are the most relevant [6, 36, 57, 58]. When treating infants, the effects of GCs on thymocyte maturation and apoptosis must also be considered [1, 8, 52]. GCs also affect dendritic cell maturation, and natural killer cell, macrophage, and neutrophil function [12, 24, 29, 32, 44, 60]. Another anti-inflammatory role of GCs is protecting cells of peripheral tissues, such as the endometrium and central nervous system [34, 54].

For these reasons, GCs remain the most potent immunosuppressive drugs available. However, GCs modulate the homeostatic functions of other cells and tissues, thus causing significant adverse effects during long-term treatment.

From a clinical point of view, although most GC therapeutic effects can last for several days or weeks after their discontinuation, they are ultimately reversible. However, a long-term benefit of GCs for patients results from the transient shutdown of inflammation, saving tissues from inflammation-derived factors. This was shown in a meta-analysis concerning radiographic progression of lesions in GC-treated patients with rheumatic disease [26]. Thus, GCs can be considered disease-modifying antirheumatic drugs.

In this chapter, we present the pharmacokinetics of old and new GCs in clinical use, as well as the mechanisms of action and innovative properties of GCs in clinical development. Moreover, we describe genetic and acquired resistance to GCs, the potential differences between responses to GCs in male and female patients, and the molecular interaction between GR and other receptors, thereby providing a rational basis for some therapeutic associations.

Past, Present, and Future GCs

Cortisol is the endogenous GC produced by the adrenal gland in significant amounts (10–20 mg) under strict control and with a circadian rhythm. Since its discovery approximately one century ago, several analogues have been synthesized. Of the GCs in clinical use, we consider old and new-generation (topical) GCs to be derivatives of cholesterol. However, within the old generation, newer GCs have some properties (particularly specificity and potency) that differ from those of cortisol and cortisone (section "Old GCs"). On the contrary, differences between the old and new generation (topical) GCs concern pharmacokinetics (section "New generation of topical GCs").

A new concept in pharmacology is biased agonism. It suggests that when a receptor activates more than one pathway, the agonist can determine which pathway is activated by the bound receptor. This idea has been demonstrated for some receptors but is likely applicable to many more. In the case of the GR, several pathways are activated, including nongenomic and genomic ones. The genomic effects include sequestration, tethering, as well as GRE and nGRE binding. Surprisingly, we know very little about the differences between old and new GCs when they bind GR, while GCs still in preclinical studies have been screened for their ability to promote GR etherodimerization but not homodimerization (section "Selective GR agonists"). Finally, new formulations of older GCs that are in clinical development may improve the concentration of GCs in target organs (section "Long-circulating liposomal GCs and other reformulations of old GCs").

Old GCs

Older-generation GCs (Table 1) are easily absorbed whether administered orally, resulting in excellent bioavailability, or topically (mucosa). GC absorption by the skin is quite effective and increases with skin inflammation, and is directly proportional to the treated surface. In emergencies, GC can be administered parenterally.

In plasma, GC binds two proteins: transcortin (also called CBG) and albumin. GCs are extensively metabolized and excreted as metabolites, some of which have weak androgenic activity. Among the old-generation GCs, the half-life tends to be longer in the newer compounds (e.g., betamethasone and dexamethasone) than in the older ones (e.g., prednisolone and triamcinolone). However, the GC half-life never exceeds 5–6 h. The duration of GC effects in target tissues (referred to as the biological half-life) is far superior to the plasma half-life owing to the genomic properties of GCs that change cell function over time. Newer GCs of the old generation are also more potent and thus can be used at lower doses. They also have much lower sodium-retention activity.

Table 1 Properties of old-generation GCs

Drug	Potency (relative to cortisol)	Salt-retaining properties	Half-life	Biologic half-life	Oral bioavailability (%)
Cortisone acetate[a]	0.8	Present	1.5	8–12	90
Prednisolone	5	Moderate	2	12–36	100
Methylprednisolone	4	Low	2.3	12–36	80–100
Triamcinolone	4	Virtually absent	1.5	12–36	100
Betamethasone	30	Virtually absent	5	36–54	90
Dexamethasone	30	Virtually absent	3.5	36–54	80–90

[a]Cortisone is a pro-drug metabolized to hydrocortisone (also called cortisol) that is the endogenous GC

New Generation of Topical GCs

New-generation GCs (Table 2) are used to treat diseases that require long-term treatment, and can also benefit local treatments. They are effective and have a decreased frequency of adverse systemic effects; therefore, new-generation GCs are the first choice for the topical treatment of asthma, allergic rhinitis, rhinosinusitis, nasal polyposis, and inflammatory bowel diseases. By contrast, old-generation GCs should not be used to treat these diseases unless systemic treatment is required owing to a lack of response to the topical treatment.

New-generation GCs can also be used in other topical treatments (e.g., eye or skin) but there is no reason to prefer them. In fact, for these treatments, the systemic side effects are infrequent and similar to those of old-generation GCs because of the low doses and the relatively low adsorption rate.

The key feature shared by all new-generation GCs is that they are much more active locally compared with the whole organism, due to pharmacokinetics properties summarized in Table 2 [15, 20, 41]. For example, studies have examined hypothalamic–pituitary–adrenal (HPA) axis suppression with intranasal GCs and have found they have minimal effects on the HPA axis [11]. The local effectiveness and systemic toxicity of inhaled GCs can be influenced by a number of drug-related systemic factors including oral bioavailability, plasma protein binding, and systemic clearance, as well as by local factors such as oral and pulmonary deposition, lipophilicity, and lipid conjugation. Local safety is influenced by the oropharyngeal deposition and activity (pro-drug vs. active drug) of the GC.

In patients with asthma, delivery devices and pharmaceutical formulations that determine particle size are crucial for increasing the percentage of GCs in the target tissue (bronchioles) and reducing the doses [47]. Inhaled GCs are generally delivered either via hydrofluoroalkane metered-dose inhalers (HFA-MDI) or dry-powder inhalers (DPI). HFA-MDI can be formulated as solutions or suspensions, and it is thought that solutions are slightly better than suspensions and DPI at delivering a greater fraction of small particles that reach the target. However, these effects depend on the drug used. Extra-fine particle formulation of HFA-beclomethasone dipropionate showed improved total and small-airway deposition as well as greater effects on lung function compared with the older large-particle chlorofluorocarbon formulation [4]. Ciclesonide has been formulated as a solution HFA-MDI with the majority of particles within the 1.1–2.1-μm size range, resulting in a very high pulmonary deposition (52 %) [19]. In order to decrease local adverse effects (dysphonia, stomatitis, and dry mouth), it is recommended to administer medication with a spacer, gargling, rinsing the mouth, and washing the face after inhalation (if nebulizers are used), as well as washing the spacer [25]. However, no scientific evidence for such procedures is available with the exception of gargling, which was shown to be protective for female patients using DPIs [35]. In children aged 2–5 years, synchronization of breathing with drug delivery is not sufficient to allow proper administration. In these patients, spacer devices with valves are indicated and are more useful than nebulizers for GC delivery, considering the importance of particle size.

Table 2 Properties of new-generation GCs

Drug name	Pro-drug	Relative potency[a] [15, 20]	Bioavailability (%) Intranasal delivery [20]	Bioavailability (%) Inhalation [15]	Biochemical properties [41] Lung deposition (pmol/g)[c]	Biochemical properties [41] Normalized lipophilicity[e]	Biochemical properties [41] Tendency to form lipid conjugates[g]	Treatment dose Allergic rhinitis (mg/day (pedex))[h]	Treatment dose Asthma (mg/day)
Beclomethasone dipropionate	Yes	13[b]	42	2 (62[b])	–[d]	–[d]	–[d]	0.08	0.3
Budesonide	No	9	33	6–13	250	1 (2,500[f])	≈100 %	0.1	0.2
Fluticasone propionate	No	8–19	2	12–17	500	3.2	0 %	0.1	0.2
Fluticasone furoate	No	30	<1	15	–[d]	–[d]	–[d]	0.05	0.2
Mometasone furoate	No	12–22	<0.1	11	150	2	0 %	0.05	0.2
Ciclesonide	Yes	12[b]	<0.1	22	180 (180[b])	4 (2.5[b])	≈50 % (≈70 %[b])	0.04	0.1

[a]As compared with dexamethasone, set equal to 1
[b]Active metabolite
[c]GC present in rat trachea following 20-min incubation with 10^{-7} M GC
[d]Not reported
[e]Normalized to budesonide
[f]Budesonide oleate
[g]Percentage of GC-ester as related to total GC present in rat trachea following 20-min incubation with 10^{-7} M GC and 3-h incubation with GC-free medium
[h]Dose per nostril

Most new-generation GCs are characterized by low bioavailability of the active drug, which is predominantly determined by four factors: significant first-pass effect, lipophilicity, strong tendency of some molecules to form lipid conjugates, and local activation (pro-drugs).

To understand the importance of the first-pass effect, it must be noted that even in the presence of an accurate delivery, the relevant percentage of an inhaled drug for asthma treatment is deposited in the mouth and first respiratory routes, and owing to mucus clearance is swallowed. A similar phenomenon is observed with GCs prescribed for allergic rhinitis treatment. Therefore, a significant first-pass effect greatly reduces the plasma concentration of the drug.

All new-generation GCs are not soluble in water with the exception of budesonide showing low water solubility. All have fairly good lipophilicity (Table 2). Moreover, budesonide and ciclesonide form esters with fatty acids (Table 2) and conjugates are pharmacologically inactive. The lipophilicity of new-generation GCs and their tendency to form lipid conjugates determine the high concentration of drug in the first cells encountered at feeding time and the slow release of active drug in the following hours. This mode of "deposit" is used to reduce the frequency and dosage of the drug, and slows drug redistribution. Moreover, beclomethasone and ciclesonide are pro-drugs that are activated more efficiently in the lung than in the oropharynx. In particular, ciclesonide is converted to the active metabolite desisobutyryl-ciclesonide (des-CIC) by esterases. Des-CIC has a much higher affinity for GR than ciclesonide has (~100 times higher) [48]. In the lung, Des-CIC forms reversible conjugates with fatty acids, such as Des-CIC oleate and Des-CIC palmitate.

New-generation GCs appear to have similar efficacies as older-generation GCs and a better safety profile. Although some pharmacological properties might suggest that mometasone and ciclesonide have a better toxicological profile compared with the other new-generation GCs, definitive data will be provided by clinical studies, particularly data assessing long-term adverse effects in children. In this context, the most interesting parameter is growth inhibition of GC-treated children with asthma. These studies are required to be performed over long periods and should provide a direct comparison between new and old GCs and how they affect growth. Moreover, growth inhibition does not necessarily become pronounced over time, but this requires even longer studies [38].

Regarding local effects, a recent study demonstrated that ciclesonide, a pro-drug, has local adverse effects similar to mometasone, which is not a pro-drug [7], suggesting that clinical translation of preclinical data is not necessarily linear. In conclusion, it is difficult at present to establish which new-generation GC should be the first choice.

Selective GR Agonists

As summarized in the preceding sections, there are several mechanisms by which GR modulates gene transcription. However, GRE-dependent transactivation and transcription factor sequestration are the most common mechanisms for promoting gene upregulation and downregulation, respectively. Because most metabolic effects of GCs depend on gene upregulation and most anti-inflammatory effects depend on decreased production of pro-inflammatory cytokines, some researchers have hypothesized that GRE-dependent transactivation is the dark side of GCs, whereas transcription factor heterodimerization and sequestration forms the basis of their anti-inflammatory activity [17, 65]. Thus, chemists have synthesized so-called selective GR agonists (SEGRAs) that favor GR heterodimerization rather than homodimerization. Such compounds, which are cholesterol-derived or nonsteroidal GCs, remain in clinical development [17, 65].

One example, 21OH-6,19OP, is a synthetic, conformationally rigid, highly bent pregnane steroid. It can bind the thymic GR but not the kidney mineral corticoid receptor or uterus progesterone receptor. It acts as a dissociated GC because it can inhibit RelA and AP-1-induced gene activation while simultaneously failing to increase liver glycogen [75]. In addition, it lacks GC-associated chemoresistance in a mouse mammary model [51].

Some dissociated GR ligands are nonsteroidal molecules, such as Abbott ligand 438 (AL-438), which possesses anti-inflammatory activity but not bone reduction in vitro, or Compound A, a plant-derived GR modulator that ameliorates clinical signs of disease in inflammatory models but with decreased side effects compared with dexamethasone [14, 16, 78].

Although some of these compounds possess anti-inflammatory properties with reduced side effects, their actual potential is still a matter of debate. The rationale on which SEGRAs are based appears to be a misinterpretation of the GC mechanism of action. Indeed, one of the pivotal mechanisms that explains the powerful anti-inflammatory effects of GCs are the very rapid, GRE-dependent upregulation of inhibitory factors, such as GILZ [3], IκB [68], annexin-1 [55], and DUSP-1 [68]. Moreover, sequestration plays a role in adverse effects. For example, RUNX2, a transcription factor crucial for osteoblastic differentiation, heterodimerizes with activated GR and is thus inhibited [40].

A deeper understanding of the molecular mechanism of action of GCs is required to dissect the pathways of GC beneficial and adverse effects, both in healthy and diseased tissues [50].

Long-Circulating Liposomal GCs and Other Reformulations of Old GCs

Another attempt to increase the therapeutic index of GCs and to target them to the site of inflammation is represented by small-sized, long-circulating liposomal GCs (less than 150 nm). These were initially formulated in topical form for dermatological purposes, but were subsequently used for intravenous administration. In this way, long-circulating liposomal GCs accumulate in ultra-high concentrations at sites of inflammation in experimental rodent models of arthritis. However, free GCs are also observed, thus causing undesirable side effects [73]. Recently, the results of the first phase I study of 22 patients with active rheumatoid arthritis (RA) who were treated with liposomal prednisolone were reported [69]. The results are encouraging and show good efficacy and safety in these patients. Clearly, further preclinical and clinical studies are necessary before determining the usefulness of small-sized long-circulating liposomal GCs.

Modifications of existing GCs can improve the daily lives of patients with RA. Morning stiffness compels these patients to take GCs during the night. New modified-release prednisone tablets have recently been developed that permit bed-time administration with programmed GC release during the night [21]. Another very recently modified GC is hydrocortisone. Under a multiparticulate oral formulation, it can mimic the diurnal cortisol profile in patients with adrenal insufficiency [76]. Loaded in nanoparticles, hydrocortisone can achieve prolonged drug release in the treatment of atopic dermatitis [62]. Thus, it is possible to modify the molecular structure or formulation of existing GCs to improve their pharmacokinetics and better treat inflammatory chronic diseases or replace endogenous hormones.

Intersubjective Variability in the Response to GCs

Genetic Resistance to GCs

GC activity depends on GR activation. Because a portion of the population fails to respond to GC treatment, studies have been conducted to identify polymorphisms in the *NR3C1* gene encoding GR.

The *Tth111*I polymorphism is located in the *NR3C1* promoter and was found to be associated with GC resistance in the presence of an ER22/23EK mutation [an arginine (R) to lysine (K) change at position 23] in exon 2. Indeed, ER22/23EK changes the tertiary structure of the GR domain, which is responsible for activation of transcription of GR mRNA. As a result, the GRα-A/GRα-B ratio changes, thereby decreasing gene transactivation. Another example is the GRβ polymorphism A3669G in the 3′-UTR of *NR3C1,* which causes an increased expression of GRβ protein owing to enhanced stability of GRβ mRNA. As explained in another chapter of this book, GRα is the fully active isoform, whereas GRβ is unable to bind any GCs and is transcriptionally inactive [27, 53]. Recently, a polymorphism in the promoter region of glucocorticoid-induced transcript-1 gene (*GLCCI1*), a protein of unknown function, was found to be correlated with reduced lung response in patients with asthma who inhaled GCs [72].

Therefore, individual heterogeneity to endogenous or exogenous GCs should be taken into account when administering GCs. Moreover, polymorphisms may be predictive of GC response, thus helping to tailor appropriate GC therapies.

Acquired Resistance to GCs

Many patients develop resistance to GC therapy during chronic inflammation, with an overall decrease in the maximum response to GCs. Because GR acts in a very complex manner and modulates expression and function of a great number of proteins, there are multiple mechanisms that can alter the pharmacological response to GCs during the development of inflammation, including different levels and function of target proteins. Moreover, the acquired resistance of inflamed tissues to GC has been postulated to correlate with a potentially low receptor reserve.

In studies in cell lines, GC resistance depended on variations in the expression of chaperone proteins such as FKBP51 and FKBP52 [64]. In patients with asthma, many molecular mechanisms correlate with GC resistance, including impaired GR nuclear translocation, decreased GR levels, increased GRβ expression, or increased AP-1 expression, which is hypothesized to impair GR function [37]. In GC refractory asthma, reduced HDAC2 expression correlates with decreased recruitment of GR to DNA sites [31]. In patients with systemic lupus erythematosus (SLE), TLR7 and TLR9 activation in plasmacytoid dendritic cells is involved in GC-induced resistance [28]. In GC-resistant ulcerative colitis, increased expression of cytokines such as tumor necrosis factor-α or interleukin-6 downregulates GR [33]. Finally, macrophage migration inhibitory factor expression has been proposed to be a common factor involved in GC-resistant inflammatory diseases, including SLE, asthma, and RA [77].

Cancer cells can be very sensitive to GC-induced apoptosis. However, they often develop resistance during chronic treatment. Some lymphoid malignancies, particularly acute lymphoblastic leukemia, can be efficiently treated with GCs because of their sensitivity to apoptosis. Because of the multiple complex mechanisms of GC action, how GCs induce apoptosis in these cells is still under investigation. One of the most recent explanations of GC resistance is site-specific phosphorylation of GR and decreased GR potency due to an altered epigenetic state in a lymphoblastic cell line. Treatment with a compound that causes DNA methylation restored GC sensitivity [46]. Other mechanisms involved in GC resistance include GR mutations and GRβ upregulation, which have been found in patients with leukemia and in cell lines. Additionally, modulation of expression of Bcl-2 family members, which are physiological targets of GCs in lymphoblasts, causes resistance to GC therapy in vivo [66].

Intracellular and extracellular signals can induce GC resistance; therefore, it is difficult to find appropriate treatments to overcome resistance once it occurs. Some attempts have been successful in preclinical studies but the complexity of GR signaling makes recovery of GC sensitivity difficult to accomplish.

GCs and Gender

GCs have recently been found to act differentially in male and female animals. In these studies, rat liver was studied as a classic target of GC action and, interestingly, unique profiles of GC-regulated genes were observed between the sexes. Among the pathways differentially altered by GC treatment in a gender-specific manner are innate immunity pathways, such as interferon or endoplasmic reticulum signaling, which account for sex-specific inflammatory stress responses. In addition, in vivo experiments showed gender-specific anti-inflammatory actions of GCs. This agrees with data showing that some chronic inflammatory autoimmune diseases (RA, SLE) occur predominantly in female patients. In addition, male and female patients respond to inflammation differently [23]. Accordingly, GC-controlled gene expression in liver is differentially regulated because GCs primarily repress genes in male and induce genes in female animals in a sexually dimorphic manner. Therefore, GC therapies should be reexamined while simultaneously taking into account that male patients respond better to anti-inflammatory treatments than their female counterparts do [59].

Molecular Basis of GC Interactions

Considering the remarkable number of effects GCs exert on various cell types in an organism, it is not surprising that molecular interactions with other drugs exist. From a clinical point of view, the most interesting is the positive interaction between GCs and β_2-agonists, and GCs and anti-muscarinic agents (section "Synergism in the treatment of asthmatic patients"). However, some interactions are deleterious, such as those observed in patients with diabetes, glaucoma, and hypertension. There are also pharmacokinetic interactions to consider (section "Pharmacokinetic interactions").

Synergism in the Treatment of Asthmatic Patients

It is well known that prolonged treatment with high doses of β_2-adrenergic agonists causes receptor desensitization. Several years ago, studies in animal models suggested that desensitization was prevented by treatment with GCs [43, 63]. In vitro studies demonstrated that GC-dependent lack of downregulation depends on the upregulation of β_2-receptors, independent of β_2-receptor triggering [43, 79]. This effect was more recently demonstrated in humans [30]. Moreover, it has been shown that β_2-adrenergic agonists can regulate GR transactivation activity by mechanisms that remain to be defined but that involve G-protein β-γ subunits and PI3-K [67].

These findings led to the evaluation of the association of β_2-adrenergic agonists and GCs in the treatment of asthma. Recently, combinations of long-acting β_2-agonists (LABAs, such as formoterol) and inhaled new topical GCs (e.g., mometasone furoate, and fluticasone) have provided definitive evidence proving the greater efficacy of combination drugs compared with the individual components in patients with asthma [9, 45].

Furthermore, the addition of a long-acting anti-muscarinic agent to an inhaled GC is as effective as LABA/GC combinations in patients with both asthma and chronic obstructive pulmonary disease [56]. In addition to clinical data, synergistic pharmacokinetic actions of LABAs and GCs have been suggested [49].

Pharmacokinetic Interactions

GCs can impact drug metabolism by altering expression of drug-metabolizing cytochromes P450 (CYPs). The mechanisms by which this occurs are complex and include regulation of CYP expression by nuclear receptors, which are directly modulated by GCs. Dexamethasone has been reported to upregulate hepatic *CYP3A1*, thus increasing *CYP3A*-dependent erythromycin demethylation [22]. In addition, GC-mediated upregulation of transcription factors such as CAR, PXR, and RXR2 and binding of activated GR to the GRE induces upregulation of *CYP2C* [10]. Moreover, *CYP2B* isozymes can be induced by GCs in liver. Variations in GC concentrations are another critical factor that either upregulates or downregulates CYP: *CYP2A* and *CYP2C* are induced at low GC concentrations but inhibited at high GC concentrations [39].

Thus, there are multiple mechanisms regulating GC control of CYP proteins, and the net response results from a combination of all factors. Understanding the molecular events underlying this control will help establish an individualized pharmacological therapy without drug–drug interactions.

Conclusions

The great novelty in the past 20 years is the development of topical GCs with increased efficacy and far fewer adverse effects. These drugs should be preferred to older GCs for the topical treatment of asthma, allergic rhinitis, rhinosinusitis, nasal polyposis, and inflammatory bowel disease. Optimization of older and newer GCs in clinical use will result from more appropriate studies regarding their mechanisms of action. For topical GCs, studies must evaluate their systemic toxicity after long-term use. New devices, solvents, and topical GC formulations will further increase their benefits and decrease their adverse effects.

The only GCs demonstrated to have biased agonism with the GR are molecules collectively called SEGRAs. They are weaker anti-inflammatory drugs but have fewer metabolic effects than the older GCs and may be useful in patients in whom the use of GCs is discouraged. Pharmacogenetic data will lead to the personalization of GC treatment and strategies to overcome GC resistance, and already offer several interesting indications.

References

1. Ashwell JD, Lu FW, Vacchio MS (2000) Glucocorticoids in T cell development and function*. Annu Rev Immunol 18:309–345. doi:10.1146/annurev.immunol.18.1.309
2. Ayroldi E, Cannarile L, Migliorati G, Nocentini G, Delfino DV, Riccardi C (2012) Mechanisms of the anti-inflammatory effects of glucocorticoids: genomic and nongenomic interference with MAPK signaling pathways. FASEB J 26(12):4805–4820. doi:10.1096/fj.12-216382
3. Ayroldi E, Riccardi C (2009) Glucocorticoid-induced leucine zipper (GILZ): a new important mediator of glucocorticoid action. FASEB J 23(11):3649–3658. doi:10.1096/fj.09-134684
4. Barnes N, Price D, Colice G, Chisholm A, Dorinsky P, Hillyer EV, Burden A, Lee AJ, Martin RJ, Roche N, von Ziegenweidt J, Israel E (2011) Asthma control with extrafine-particle hydrofluoroalkane-beclometasone vs. large-particle chlorofluorocarbon-beclometasone: a real-world observational study. Clin Exp Allergy 41(11):1521–1532. doi:10.1111/j.1365-2222.2011.03820.x
5. Beck IM, Vanden Berghe W, Vermeulen L, Yamamoto KR, Haegeman G, De Bosscher K (2009) Crosstalk in inflammation: the interplay of glucocorticoid receptor-based mechanisms and kinases and phosphatases. Endocr Rev 30(7):830–882. doi:10.1210/er.2009-0013
6. Bereshchenko O, Coppo M, Bruscoli S, Biagioli M, Cimino M, Frammartino T, Sorcini D, Venanzi A, Di Sante M, Riccardi C (2014) GILZ promotes production of peripherally induced treg cells and mediates the crosstalk between glucocorticoids and TGF-beta signaling. Cell Rep 7(2):464–475. doi:10.1016/j.celrep.2014.03.004
7. Berger WE, Prenner B, Turner R, Meltzer EO (2013) A patient preference and satisfaction study of ciclesonide nasal aerosol and mometasone furoate aqueous nasal spray in patients with perennial allergic rhinitis. Allergy Asthma Proc 34(6):542–550. doi:10.2500/aap.2013.34.3705
8. Bianchini R, Nocentini G, Krausz LT, Fettucciari K, Coaccioli S, Ronchetti S, Riccardi C (2006) Modulation of pro- and antiapoptotic molecules in double-positive (CD4+CD8+) thymocytes following dexamethasone treatment. J Pharmacol Exp Ther 319(2):887–897. doi:10.1124/jpet.106.108480
9. Bodzenta-Lukaszyk A, Dymek A, McAulay K, Mansikka H (2011) Fluticasone/formoterol combination therapy is as effective as fluticasone/salmeterol in the treatment of asthma, but has a more rapid onset of action: an open-label, randomized study. BMC Pulm Med 11:28. doi:10.1186/1471-2466-11-28
10. Brtko J, Dvorak Z (2011) Role of retinoids, rexinoids and thyroid hormone in the expression of cytochrome p450 enzymes. Curr Drug Metab 12(2):71–88
11. Bruni FM, De Luca G, Venturoli V, Boner AL (2009) Intranasal corticosteroids and adrenal suppression. Neuroimmunomodulation 16(5):353–362. doi:10.1159/000216193
12. Bush KA, Krukowski K, Eddy JL, Janusek LW, Mathews HL (2012) Glucocorticoid receptor mediated suppression of natural killer cell activity: identification of associated deacetylase and corepressor molecules. Cell Immunol 275(1–2):80–89. doi:10.1016/j.cellimm.2012.02.014
13. Busillo JM, Cidlowski JA (2013) The five Rs of glucocorticoid action during inflammation: ready, reinforce, repress, resolve, and restore. Trends Endocrinol Metab 24(3):109–119. doi:10.1016/j.tem.2012.11.005
14. Coghlan MJ, Jacobson PB, Lane B, Nakane M, Lin CW, Elmore SW, Kym PR, Luly JR, Carter GW, Turner R, Tyree CM, Hu J, Elgort M, Rosen J, Miner JN (2003) A novel antiinflammatory maintains glucocorticoid efficacy with reduced side effects. Mol Endocrinol 17(5):860–869. doi:10.1210/me.2002-0355
15. Crim C, Pierre LN, Daley-Yates PT (2001) A review of the pharmacology and pharmacokinetics of inhaled fluticasone propionate and mometasone furoate. Clin Ther 23(9):1339–1354
16. De Bosscher K, Beck IM, Haegeman G (2010) Classic glucocorticoids versus non-steroidal glucocorticoid receptor modulators: survival of the fittest regulator of the immune system? Brain Behav Immun 24(7):1035–1042. doi:10.1016/j.bbi.2010.06.010

17. De Bosscher K, Haegeman G (2009) Minireview: latest perspectives on antiinflammatory actions of glucocorticoids. Mol Endocrinol 23(3):281–291. doi:10.1210/me.2008-0283
18. De Bosscher K, Vanden Berghe W, Haegeman G (2006) Cross-talk between nuclear receptors and nuclear factor kappaB. Oncogene 25(51):6868–6886. doi:10.1038/sj.onc.1209935
19. Derendorf H (2007) Pharmacokinetic and pharmacodynamic properties of inhaled ciclesonide. J Clin Pharmacol 47(6):782–789. doi:10.1177/0091270007299763
20. Derendorf H, Meltzer EO (2008) Molecular and clinical pharmacology of intranasal corticosteroids: clinical and therapeutic implications. Allergy 63(10):1292–1300. doi:10.1111/j.1398-9995.2008.01750.x
21. Derendorf H, Ruebsamen K, Clarke L, Schaeffler A, Kirwan JR (2013) Pharmacokinetics of modified-release prednisone tablets in healthy subjects and patients with rheumatoid arthritis. J Clin Pharmacol 53(3):326–333. doi:10.1177/0091270012444315
22. Dey A, Yadav S, Dhawan A, Seth PK, Parmar D (2006) Evidence for cytochrome P450 3A expression and catalytic activity in rat blood lymphocytes. Life Sci 79(18):1729–1735. doi:10.1016/j.lfs.2006.06.006
23. Duma D, Collins JB, Chou JW, Cidlowski JA (2010) Sexually dimorphic actions of glucocorticoids provide a link to inflammatory diseases with gender differences in prevalence. Sci Signal 3(143):ra74. doi:10.1126/scisignal.2001077
24. Ehrchen J, Steinmuller L, Barczyk K, Tenbrock K, Nacken W, Eisenacher M, Nordhues U, Sorg C, Sunderkotter C, Roth J (2007) Glucocorticoids induce differentiation of a specifically activated, anti-inflammatory subtype of human monocytes. Blood 109(3):1265–1274. doi:10.1182/blood-2006-02-001115
25. Galvan CA, Guarderas JC (2012) Practical considerations for dysphonia caused by inhaled corticosteroids. Mayo Clin Proc 87(9):901–904. doi:10.1016/j.mayocp.2012.06.022
26. Graudal N, Jurgens G (2010) Similar effects of disease-modifying antirheumatic drugs, glucocorticoids, and biologic agents on radiographic progression in rheumatoid arthritis: meta-analysis of 70 randomized placebo-controlled or drug-controlled studies, including 112 comparisons. Arthritis Rheum 62(10):2852–2863. doi:10.1002/art.27592
27. Gross KL, Cidlowski JA (2008) Tissue-specific glucocorticoid action: a family affair. Trends Endocrinol Metab 19(9):331–339. doi:10.1016/j.tem.2008.07.009
28. Guiducci C, Gong M, Xu Z, Gill M, Chaussabel D, Meeker T, Chan JH, Wright T, Punaro M, Bolland S, Soumelis V, Banchereau J, Coffman RL, Pascual V, Barrat FJ (2010) TLR recognition of self nucleic acids hampers glucocorticoid activity in lupus. Nature 465(7300):937–941. doi:10.1038/nature09102
29. Hamdi H, Godot V, Maillot MC, Prejean MV, Cohen N, Krzysiek R, Lemoine FM, Zou W, Emilie D (2007) Induction of antigen-specific regulatory T lymphocytes by human dendritic cells expressing the glucocorticoid-induced leucine zipper. Blood 110(1):211–219. doi:10.1182/blood-2006-10-052506
30. Hauck RW, Harth M, Schulz C, Prauer H, Bohm M, Schomig A (1997) Effects of beta 2-agonist- and dexamethasone-treatment on relaxation and regulation of beta-adrenoceptors in human bronchi and lung tissue. Br J Pharmacol 121(8):1523–1530. doi:10.1038/sj.bjp.0701289
31. Hew M, Bhavsar P, Torrego A, Meah S, Khorasani N, Barnes PJ, Adcock I, Chung KF (2006) Relative corticosteroid insensitivity of peripheral blood mononuclear cells in severe asthma. Am J Respir Crit Care Med 174(2):134–141. doi:10.1164/rccm.200512-1930OC
32. Hirsch G, Lavoie-Lamoureux A, Beauchamp G, Lavoie JP (2012) Neutrophils are not less sensitive than other blood leukocytes to the genomic effects of glucocorticoids. PLoS One 7(9):e44606. doi:10.1371/journal.pone.0044606
33. Ishiguro Y (1999) Mucosal proinflammatory cytokine production correlates with endoscopic activity of ulcerative colitis. J Gastroenterol 34(1):66–74
34. Jing Y, Hou Y, Song Y, Yin J (2012) Methylprednisolone improves the survival of new neurons following transient cerebral ischemia in rats. Acta Neurobiol Exp 72(3):240–252
35. Kajiwara A, Kita A, Saruwatari J, Morita K, Oniki K, Yamamura M, Murase M, Koda H, Hirota S, Ishizuka T, Nakagawa K (2014) Absence of gargling affects topical adverse

symptoms caused by inhaled corticosteroids in females. J Asthma 51(2):221–224. doi:10.3109/02770903.2013.857683

36. Karagiannidis C, Akdis M, Holopainen P, Woolley NJ, Hense G, Ruckert B, Mantel PY, Menz G, Akdis CA, Blaser K, Schmidt-Weber CB (2004) Glucocorticoids upregulate FOXP3 expression and regulatory T cells in asthma. J Allergy Clin Immunol 114(6):1425–1433. doi:10.1016/j.jaci.2004.07.014
37. Keenan CR, Salem S, Fietz ER, Gualano RC, Stewart AG (2012) Glucocorticoid-resistant asthma and novel anti-inflammatory drugs. Drug Discov Today 17(17–18):1031–1038. doi:10.1016/j.drudis.2012.05.011
38. Kelly HW, Sternberg AL, Lescher R, Fuhlbrigge AL, Williams P, Zeiger RS, Raissy HH, Van Natta ML, Tonascia J, Strunk RC, CAMP Research Group (2012) Effect of inhaled glucocorticoids in childhood on adult height. N Engl J Med 367(10):904–912. doi:10.1056/NEJMoa1203229
39. Konstandi M, Johnson EO, Lang MA (2014) Consequences of psychophysiological stress on cytochrome P450-catalyzed drug metabolism. Neurosci Biobehav Rev 45C:149–167. doi:10.1016/j.neubiorev.2014.05.011
40. Koromila T, Baniwal SK, Song YS, Martin A, Xiong J, Frenkel B (2014) Glucocorticoids antagonize RUNX2 during osteoblast differentiation in cultures of ST2 pluripotent mesenchymal cells. J Cell Biochem 115(1):27–33. doi:10.1002/jcb.24646
41. Lexmuller K, Gullstrand H, Axelsson BO, Sjolin P, Korn SH, Silberstein DS, Miller-Larsson A (2007) Differences in endogenous esterification and retention in the rat trachea between budesonide and ciclesonide active metabolite. Drug Metab Dispos 35(10):1788–1796. doi:10.1124/dmd.107.015297
42. Liberman AC, Refojo D, Druker J, Toscano M, Rein T, Holsboer F, Arzt E (2007) The activated glucocorticoid receptor inhibits the transcription factor T-bet by direct protein-protein interaction. FASEB J 21(4):1177–1188. doi:10.1096/fj.06-7452com
43. Mak JC, Nishikawa M, Shirasaki H, Miyayasu K, Barnes PJ (1995) Protective effects of a glucocorticoid on downregulation of pulmonary beta 2-adrenergic receptors in vivo. J Clin Invest 96(1):99–106. doi:10.1172/JCI118084
44. Matyszak MK, Citterio S, Rescigno M, Ricciardi-Castagnoli P (2000) Differential effects of corticosteroids during different stages of dendritic cell maturation. Eur J Immunol 30(4):1233–1242. doi:10.1002/(SICI)1521-4141(200004)30:4<1233::AID-IMMU1233>3.0.CO;2-F
45. Meltzer EO, Kuna P, Nolte H, Nayak AS, Laforce C, Investigators PS (2012) Mometasone furoate/formoterol reduces asthma deteriorations and improves lung function. Eur Respir J 39(2):279–289. doi:10.1183/09031936.00020310
46. Miller AL, Geng C, Golovko G, Sharma M, Schwartz JR, Yan J, Sowers L, Widger WR, Fofanov Y, Vedeckis WV, Thompson EB (2014) Epigenetic alteration by DNA-demethylating treatment restores apoptotic response to glucocorticoids in dexamethasone-resistant human malignant lymphoid cells. Cancer Cell Int 14:35. doi:10.1186/1475-2867-14-35
47. Muller V, Galffy G, Eszes N, Losonczy G, Bizzi A, Nicolini G, Chrystyn H, Tamasi L (2011) Asthma control in patients receiving inhaled corticosteroid and long-acting beta2-agonist fixed combinations. A real-life study comparing dry powder inhalers and a pressurized metered dose inhaler extrafine formulation. BMC Pulm Med 11:40. doi:10.1186/1471-2466-11-40
48. Nave R, Watz H, Hoffmann H, Boss H, Magnussen H (2010) Deposition and metabolism of inhaled ciclesonide in the human lung. Eur Respir J 36(5):1113–1119. doi:10.1183/09031936.00172309
49. Nie M, Corbett L, Knox AJ, Pang L (2005) Differential regulation of chemokine expression by peroxisome proliferator-activated receptor gamma agonists: interactions with glucocorticoids and beta2-agonists. J Biol Chem 280(4):2550–2561. doi:10.1074/jbc.M410616200
50. Oakley RH, Cidlowski JA (2013) The biology of the glucocorticoid receptor: new signaling mechanisms in health and disease. J Allergy Clin Immunol 132(5):1033–1044. doi:10.1016/j.jaci.2013.09.007
51. Orqueda AJ, Dansey MV, Espanol A, Veleiro AS, de Kier B, Joffe E, Sales ME, Burton G, Pecci A (2014) The rigid steroid 21-hydroxy-6,19-epoxyprogesterone (21OH-6,19OP) is a

dissociated glucocorticoid receptor modulator potentially useful as a novel coadjuvant in breast cancer chemotherapy. Biochem Pharmacol 89(4):526–535. doi:10.1016/j.bcp.2014.04.006
52. Palinkas L, Talaber G, Boldizsar F, Bartis D, Nemeth P, Berki T (2008) Developmental shift in TcR-mediated rescue of thymocytes from glucocorticoid-induced apoptosis. Immunobiology 213(1):39–50. doi:10.1016/j.imbio.2007.06.004
53. Panek M, Pietras T, Fabijan A, Milanowski M, Wieteska L, Gorski P, Kuna P, Szemraj J (2013) Effect of glucocorticoid receptor gene polymorphisms on asthma phenotypes. Exp Ther Med 5(2):572–580. doi:10.3892/etm.2012.809
54. Pecci A, Scholz A, Pelster D, Beato M (1997) Progestins prevent apoptosis in a rat endometrial cell line and increase the ratio of bcl-XL to bcl-XS. J Biol Chem 272(18):11791–11798
55. Perretti M, D'Acquisto F (2009) Annexin A1 and glucocorticoids as effectors of the resolution of inflammation. Nat Rev Immunol 9(1):62–70. doi:10.1038/nri2470
56. Peters SP, Kunselman SJ, Icitovic N, Moore WC, Pascual R, Ameredes BT, Boushey HA, Calhoun WJ, Castro M, Cherniack RM, Craig T, Denlinger L, Engle LL, DiMango EA, Fahy JV, Israel E, Jarjour N, Kazani SD, Kraft M, Lazarus SC, Lemanske RF Jr, Lugogo N, Martin RJ, Meyers DA, Ramsdell J, Sorkness CA, Sutherland ER, Szefler SJ, Wasserman SI, Walter MJ, Wechsler ME, Chinchilli VM, Bleecker ER, National Heart, Lung, and Blood Institute Asthma Clinical Research Network (2010) Tiotropium bromide step-up therapy for adults with uncontrolled asthma. N Engl J Med 363(18):1715–1726. doi:10.1056/NEJMoa1008770
57. Petrillo MG, Fettucciari K, Montuschi P, Ronchetti S, Cari L, Migliorati G, Mazzon E, Bereshchenko O, Bruscoli S, Nocentini G, Riccardi C (2014) Transcriptional regulation of kinases downstream of the T cell receptor: another immunomodulatory mechanism of glucocorticoids. BMC Pharmacol Toxicol 15:35. doi:10.1186/2050-6511-15-35
58. Prado C, Gomez J, Lopez P, de Paz B, Gutierrez C, Suarez A (2011) Dexamethasone upregulates FOXP3 expression without increasing regulatory activity. Immunobiology 216(3):386–392. doi:10.1016/j.imbio.2010.06.013
59. Quinn M, Ramamoorthy S, Cidlowski JA (2014) Sexually dimorphic actions of glucocorticoids: beyond chromosomes and sex hormones. Ann N Y Acad Sci 1317:1–6. doi:10.1111/nyas.12425
60. Riccardi C, Bruscoli S, Ayroldi E, Agostini M, Migliorati G (2001) GILZ, a glucocorticoid hormone induced gene, modulates T lymphocytes activation and death through interaction with NF-kB. Adv Exp Med Biol 495:31–39
61. Ronchetti S, Migliorati G, Riccardi C (2014) Glucocorticoid-Induced Immunomodulation. In: Corsini E, van Loveren H, (eds); Wiley Blackwell, Weinheim, Germany. pp. 209–226. doi:10.1002/9783527676965.ch10
62. Rosado C, Silva C, Reis CP (2013) Hydrocortisone-loaded poly(epsilon-caprolactone) nanoparticles for atopic dermatitis treatment. Pharm Dev Technol 18(3):710–718. doi:10.3109/10837450.2012.712537
63. Salonen RO (1985) Concomitant glucocorticoid treatment prevents the development of beta-adrenoceptor desensitization in the guinea pig lung. Acta Pharmacol Toxicol 57(3):147–153
64. Scammell JG, Denny WB, Valentine DL, Smith DF (2001) Overexpression of the FK506-binding immunophilin FKBP51 is the common cause of glucocorticoid resistance in three New World primates. Gen Comp Endocrinol 124(2):152–165. doi:10.1006/gcen.2001.7696
65. Schacke H, Berger M, Rehwinkel H, Asadullah K (2007) Selective glucocorticoid receptor agonists (SEGRAs): novel ligands with an improved therapeutic index. Mol Cell Endocrinol 275(1–2):109–117. doi:10.1016/j.mce.2007.05.014
66. Schlossmacher G, Stevens A, White A (2011) Glucocorticoid receptor-mediated apoptosis: mechanisms of resistance in cancer cells. J Endocrinol 211(1):17–25. doi:10.1530/JOE-11-0135
67. Schmidt P, Holsboer F, Spengler D (2001) Beta(2)-adrenergic receptors potentiate glucocorticoid receptor transactivation via G protein beta gamma-subunits and the phosphoinositide 3-kinase pathway. Mol Endocrinol 15(4):553–564. doi:10.1210/mend.15.4.0613
68. Shipp LE, Lee JV, Yu CY, Pufall M, Zhang P, Scott DK, Wang JC (2010) Transcriptional regulation of human dual specificity protein phosphatase 1 (DUSP1) gene by glucocorticoids. PLoS One 5(10):e13754. doi:10.1371/journal.pone.0013754

69. Spies CM, Bijlsma JW, Burmester GR, Buttgereit F (2010) Pharmacology of glucocorticoids in rheumatoid arthritis. Curr Opin Pharmacol 10(3):302–307. doi:10.1016/j.coph.2010.02.001
70. Strehl C, Buttgereit F (2014) Unraveling the functions of the membrane-bound glucocorticoid receptors: first clues on origin and functional activity. Ann N Y Acad Sci 1318(1):1–6. doi:10.1111/nyas.12364
71. Surjit M, Ganti KP, Mukherji A, Ye T, Hua G, Metzger D, Li M, Chambon P (2011) Widespread negative response elements mediate direct repression by agonist-liganded glucocorticoid receptor. Cell 145(2):224–241. doi:10.1016/j.cell.2011.03.027
72. Tantisira KG, Lasky-Su J, Harada M, Murphy A, Litonjua AA, Himes BE, Lange C, Lazarus R, Sylvia J, Klanderman B, Duan QL, Qiu W, Hirota T, Martinez FD, Mauger D, Sorkness C, Szefler S, Lazarus SC, Lemanske RF Jr, Peters SP, Lima JJ, Nakamura Y, Tamari M, Weiss ST (2011) Genomewide association between GLCCI1 and response to glucocorticoid therapy in asthma. N Engl J Med 365(13):1173–1183. doi:10.1056/NEJMoa0911353
73. van den Hoven JM, Hofkens W, Wauben MH, Wagenaar-Hilbers JP, Beijnen JH, Nuijen B, Metselaar JM, Storm G (2011) Optimizing the therapeutic index of liposomal glucocorticoids in experimental arthritis. Int J Pharm 416(2):471–477. doi:10.1016/j.ijpharm.2011.03.025
74. Vandevyver S, Dejager L, Tuckermann J, Libert C (2013) New insights into the anti-inflammatory mechanisms of glucocorticoids: an emerging role for glucocorticoid-receptor-mediated transactivation. Endocrinology 154(3):993–1007. doi:10.1210/en.2012-2045
75. Vicent GP, Monteserin MC, Veleiro AS, Burton G, Lantos CP, Galigniana MD (1997) 21-Hydroxy-6,19-oxidoprogesterone: a novel synthetic steroid with specific antiglucocorticoid properties in the rat. Mol Pharmacol 52(4):749–753
76. Whitaker MJ, Debono M, Huatan H, Merke DP, Arlt W, Ross RJ (2014) An oral multiparticulate, modified-release, hydrocortisone replacement therapy that provides physiological cortisol exposure. Clin Endocrinol (Oxf) 80(4):554–561. doi:10.1111/cen.12316
77. Yang N, Ray DW, Matthews LC (2012) Current concepts in glucocorticoid resistance. Steroids 77(11):1041–1049. doi:10.1016/j.steroids.2012.05.007
78. Zhang Z, Zhang ZY, Schluesener HJ (2009) Compound A, a plant origin ligand of glucocorticoid receptors, increases regulatory T cells and M2 macrophages to attenuate experimental autoimmune neuritis with reduced side effects. J Immunol 183(5):3081–3091. doi:10.4049/jimmunol.0901088
79. Zhong H, Minneman KP (1993) Close reciprocal regulation of beta 1- and beta 2-adrenergic receptors by dexamethasone in C6 glioma cells: effects on catecholamine responsiveness. Mol Pharmacol 44(6):1085–1093

Corticosteroids in Juvenile Idiopathic Arthritis

María M. Katsicas and Ricardo A.G. Russo

The Use of Corticosteroids in the Treatment of Juvenile Idiopathic Arthritis

Juvenile idiopathic arthritis (JIA) is the most common chronic rheumatic condition of childhood and an important cause of disability and poor quality of life [1]. JIA is defined as chronic, idiopathic arthritis occurring in an individual younger than 16 years of age, but it is likely not a single disease. It is an umbrella term for a group of related – albeit heterogeneous – disorders characterized by chronic arthritis (and involvement of other organs). The cause of JIA is not known, but there is ample evidence of the participation of different genetic, environmental, and immunological factors in its pathogenesis [2]. The International League of Associations for Rheumatology proposed a classification of the different idiopathic arthritides of childhood [3]. This classification has allowed for the inclusion of patients with JIA in fairly homogeneous, well-defined disease categories thus benefitting international communication and research. In the International League of Associations for Rheumatology classification, JIA is categorized into seven groups that may well represent different diseases: systemic arthritis, rheumatoid factor–positive polyarthritis, rheumatoid factor–negative polyarthritis, oligoarthritis, psoriatic arthritis, enthesitis-related arthritis (ERA; comprising the majority of patients with juvenile spondyloarthropathy), and undifferentiated arthritis (Table 1). These mutually exclusive groups are defined by unique clinical, immunological, and immunogenetic features.

Corticosteroids have been used for the treatment of JIA since the 1950s [4]. New, effective, and safe biological therapies have revolutionized the management of JIA

M.M. Katsicas, MD (✉) • R.A.G. Russo, MD
Service of Immunology and Rheumatology, Hospital de Pediatría "Prof. Dr. Juan P. Garrahan", Pichincha 1880, Buenos Aires 1245, Argentina
e-mail: mmkatsi@yahoo.com.ar; rrusso@garrahan.gov.ar

R. Cimaz (ed.), *Systemic Corticosteroids for Inflammatory Disorders in Pediatrics*, DOI 10.1007/978-3-319-16056-6_6

Table 1 International League of Associations for Rheumatology JIA classification [2]

Category	Definition	Exclusions
Systemic	Arthritis in one or more joints with or preceded by fever of at least 2-week duration. Signs or symptoms must have been documented daily for at least 3 days and accompanied by one or more of the following: evanescent rash, generalized lymphadenopathy, hepatomegaly, serositis.	A, B, C, D
Persistent or extended oligoarthritis	Arthritis affecting one to four joints during the first 6 months. Persistent oligoarthritis affects up to four joints throughout the course of the disease, and extended oligoarthritis affects more than four joints after the first 6 months.	A, B, C, D, E
RF-negative polyarthritis	Rheumatoid factor-negative arthritis affecting five or more joints during the first 6 months of disease.	A, B, C, D, E
RF-positive polyarthritis	There is rheumatoid factor-negative arthritis affecting five or more joints during the first 6 months of disease. Two or more RF tests (taken at least 3 months apart) are positive during the first 6 months of disease.	A, B, C, E
Psoriatic	Arthritis and psoriasis or arthritis with at least two of the following: dactylitis, nail pitting, onycholysis, and/or family history of psoriasis (in a first-degree relative).	B, C, D, E
Enthesitis-related arthritis	Arthritis and/or enteritis with at least two of the following: presence of history of sacroiliac joint tenderness with or without inflammatory lumbosacral pain, presence of HLA-B27 antigen, onset of arthritis in a male patient over 6 years of age, acute (symptomatic) anterior uveitis, history of ankylosing spondylitis, enthesitis-related arthritis, sacroiliitis with inflammatory bowel disease, Reiter's syndrome, or acute anterior uveitis in a first-degree relative.	A, D, E
Undifferentiated	Arthritis that does not fulfill criteria in any of the above categories or that fulfills criteria for two or more of the above categories.	

Exclusions

A: Psoriasis or history of psoriasis in patients or first-degree relatives

B: Arthritis in HLA-B27-positive male patients beginning after the age of 6 years

C: Ankylosing spondylitis, enthesitis-related arthritis, sacroiliitis with inflammatory bowel disease, Reiter's syndrome, acute anterior uveitis, or history of one of these disorders in first-degree relatives

D: Presence of IgM rheumatoid factor on at least two occasions at least 3 months apart

E: Presence of systemic JIA in patients

in the past few years [5–9], but corticosteroids still have their place in the pharmacological therapy of these diseases. Owing to a lack of controlled studies of the use of corticosteroids in JIA, treatment has usually been supported by level 4 or 5 evidence (expert opinion or descriptive studies). In the past few years, the elaboration of clinical guidelines and consensus statements has added important tools to the management of steroids in children with JIA.

The indication of corticosteroids is somewhat different for each JIA category. As a general rule, systemic corticosteroids are prescribed to treat patients with systemic JIA who exhibit extra-articular features such as refractory anemia, serositis, and the macrophage activation syndrome (MAS). The presence of fever or arthritis alone is not an indication for systemic corticosteroid therapy in any form of JIA. On the other hand, low-dose, short-term systemic corticosteroids may be indicated in severe forms of polyarthritis or ERA and for chronic JIA-related uveitis refractory to local therapy.

Different corticosteroid agents have been used for the systemic treatment of JIA: Prednisone, prednisolone, methylprednisolone, and deflazacort are the most frequently used drugs. The disease-modifying effect of glucocorticoids is mostly related to anti-inflammatory actions such as inhibition of interleukin (IL)-1 and IL-6, as well as suppression of proinflammatory mediators such as eicosanoids and reactive oxygen species [10]. Prednisone is the most widely used corticosteroid in the treatment of JIA. In the 1990s, deflazacort became an alternative corticosteroid for systemic use because of its presumed bone-sparing properties as compared with prednisone [11]. In one study, a small cohort of patients with JIA treated with deflazacort showed an advantage over prednisone. Children showed significant lumbar bone loss only in the prednisone group [12]. However, its clinical use was short-lived and prednisone (or methylprednisone) has remained the most frequently used and recommended corticosteroid agent [13].

The use of continuous, higher-dose corticosteroids is not devoid of adverse events. The use of intermittent intravenous higher-dose steroids ("pulse therapy") has shown to be safer than continuous, oral treatment, supposedly due to the lower cumulative dose needed to control JIA inflammatory activity [14, 15]. The effect of corticosteroid therapy over linear growth in patients with JIA has long been recognized [4]. Prolonged use of systemic corticosteroids may cause reduction in bone mineral density and vertebral fractures [16, 17] and growth impairment [18, 19] in patients with JIA. Patients with a systemic onset or polyarticular course (who require more intense and more prolonged corticosteroid therapy) are at a higher risk of corticosteroid-related adverse events. Simon et al. found a significant loss of height during the first years of the disease course in a cohort of patients with JIA who had been treated with systemic corticosteroids. In this study, loss of height correlated with the duration of prednisone therapy [20]. These authors also found that 30 % of the patients did not achieve a catch-up growth. An alternate-day regimen may decrease the deleterious effect of corticosteroids on height velocity [21]. Finally, the use of systemic corticosteroids may negatively influence the nutritional status of children with JIA by increasing body mass index, particularly in patients with systemic JIA [22, 23].

Corticosteroids in the Different JIA Categories

Evidence shows that systemic corticosteroids are widely used in all types of JIA, more often in systemic JIA. Recent surveys indicated that systemic corticosteroids are used in over 80 % of patients with systemic JIA, and over 35 % of all patients with any type of JIA. In the United States, the ever-use of systemic corticosteroids was reported to be 83 % for patients with systemic JIA, 63 % for rheumatoid factor–positive polyarthritis, 42 % for rheumatoid factor-negative polyarthritis, 36 % for ERA, 35 % for undifferentiated arthritis, 33 % for psoriatic arthritis, 27 % for extended oligoarthritis, and 16 % for persistent oligoarthritis [13]. A comparative analysis of two health-care systems showed German/Austrian and Canadian treating physicians prescribed systemic corticosteroids in 19–34 % of polyarthritis cases, while intra-articular corticosteroid therapy was more frequent for both oligoarthritis and polyarthritis in both settings. In this analysis, the European groups appeared to be more prone to using steroids in all JIA groups [24]. Nevertheless, the more frequent use of new therapies (such as anakinra, canakinumab, and tocilizumab) is leading to such agents being used at a lower rate [25, 26].

Systemic JIA

Systemic corticosteroids are frequently used in the treatment of systemic JIA [26]. However, new, effective, and safe biologic agents have been introduced to the treatment of systemic JIA in the past few years, and hopefully will change the short- and long-term course of the disease. The IL-1-blocking agents anakinra [7] and canakinumab [6] and the IL-6R antagonist tocilizumab [5] have added a completely new paradigm in the treatment of systemic JIA.

The indications for systemic corticosteroids in systemic JIA have traditionally been serositis (pleuritis, peritonitis, or pericarditis), myocarditis or evidence of MAS, in which high doses [prednisone 1–2 mg/kg per day or pulse intravenous methylprednisolone (30 mg/kg per day) for 3 days] are needed for rapid control of systemic features [27–32]. After pulse steroids, daily prednisone at 2 mg/kg per day may be initiated with gradual tapering once inactive disease is achieved. In 1996 Picco et al. published their experience with corticosteroid "minipulses" [14]. The authors used methylprednisolone 5 mg/kg per day for 3 days with an additional course of methylprednisolone 2.5 mg/kg per day for 3 days, followed by prednisone 1 mg/kg daily in 12 patients with systemic JIA. Patients had a remarkable improvement in articular, systemic, and hematologic features as compared with ten patients who received prednisone 1 mg/kg per day. Patients receiving pulse steroids may exhibit side effects (such as behavioral changes, headaches, hypertension, tachycardia, and abdominal pain) [15, 30] but they require a lower cumulative daily dosage than conventional oral corticosteroid treatment. In the 1990s, aggressive combined therapy including cyclophosphamide, methotrexate (MTX), and pulse therapy with methylprednisolone was advocated for systemic arthritis [31, 32]. With the advent of biological agents in the beginning of the following decade, these approaches were abandoned or restricted to exceptionally refractory cases. On the other hand, low-dose systemic corticosteroid therapy may be useful for minor disease features, such as anemia of inflammatory disease, persistent activity despite the use of nonsteroidal anti-inflammatory drugs (NSAIDs), and bridging to biological therapy. These indications are relative and are usually tailored for each individual by the treating physician.

Owing to the high variability in therapeutic approaches and corticosteroid usage among different groups, several efforts have been made to standardize corticosteroid therapy in systemic JIA. Recently, a group of experts defined the management of background corticosteroid therapy in clinical trials in systemic JIA that could be adopted for clinical ordinary practice [33]. These investigators identified criteria for initiating or increasing corticosteroids such as presence or development of anemia (with hemoglobin <6.5 g/dl), symptomatic myocarditis, pericarditis, pleuritis, peritonitis, pneumonitis, and either complete or incomplete MAS. The presence of fever, rash, severe fatigue, anorexia, weight loss, increasing synovitis, and low albumin did not represent criteria for initiating or increasing corticosteroids. For MAS, pericarditis, and myocarditis, they defined a corticosteroid therapy approach comprising high-dose intravenous methylprednisolone pulse (30 mg/kg/day for 1–3 days) followed by daily standard-dose corticosteroids. The rate of taper of corticosteroid dosing was defined as 10 % of the current daily dose every 2 weeks.

Another consensus meeting generated a treatment approach that offered among four treatment plans (corticosteroids alone, MTX, anakinra, or tocilizumab) a choice of either high-dose (2 mg/kg/daily) or low-dose (0.5 mg/kg/daily) oral prednisone, with methylprednisolone pulses and/or intra-articular injections as needed for patients with systemic JIA [25]. According to this consensus, the goal was to discontinue glucocorticoids by 6 months, with three defined tapering schedules (rapid, fast, and slow) to proceed as tolerated. One suggested treatment plan included corticosteroids only [prednisone 1 mg/kg per day (maximum 60 mg), with optional use of methylprednisolone pulse (30 mg/kg, max. 1 g for 3 days)]. According to the clinical status of the patient at 1–2 weeks, at 1 month and at 3 months the corticosteroid dosing could be tapered, increased to 2 mg/kg (maximum 100 mg) daily, or kept with no changes. In case of improvement, the consensus agreed that corticosteroid dosage should be tapered and total treatment with corticosteroids should not last more than 6 months. Prednisone was also included as an optional therapy in the MTX, anti-IL-1, and anti-IL-6 plans.

The American College of Rheumatology (ACR) elaborated and recently revised the recommendations for the treatment of JIA [34, 35]. In the original recommendations [34], two categories were considered for systemic JIA: patients with systemic features and patients with active arthritis. Introduction of systemic corticosteroids was recommended after the unsuccessful use of NSAIDs for 2 weeks, or earlier for patients with persistent fever or higher disease activity (MD global ≥7). The 2013 revision of these guidelines provided an expanded recommendation on the use of corticosteroids and other agents in the treatment of systemic JIA [35]. For patients with active systemic features and varying degrees of synovitis, systemic corticosteroid monotherapy (either oral or intravenous) was recommended for a maximum period of 2 weeks, with an evidence level 3. Continuing corticosteroids as monotherapy for more than 1 month for patients with continued disease activity was considered inappropriate (level 4). For this same group of patients, anakinra was recommended as an initial therapeutic option. For systemic JIA without active systemic features and active synovitis, corticosteroids were recommended only as intra-articular therapy at any time. However, the utility of repeating intra-articular injection as the only intervention was considered uncertain. Since the efficacy of intra-articular corticosteroid therapy in systemic JIA is usually shorter than the one observed in other forms of JIA [36–40], this approach should probably be limited to special situations (quick relief of pain or dysfunction) [41]. Additional recommendations were made for patients with systemic JIA and features suggestive of MAS. These recommendations are described in the next sections.

A summary of the different studies on the use of systemic corticosteroids in systemic JIA is given in Table 2.

Polyarticular JIA

Systemic corticosteroids are not the mainstay of therapy in polyarticular JIA (rheumatoid factor-positive or -negative). However, systemic corticosteroids are frequently used as bridging therapy in low doses (0.1–0.2 mg/kg per day) and short periods to help ameliorate the inflammatory features until the background medications (MTX or biologics) are effective. This strategy is useful for reaching an earlier resolution of synovitis as well as improvement in functional capacity and quality of life [29].

An "aggressive" approach to the initial therapy of polyarticular JIA was recently published by Wallace et al. [42]. It included prednisolone, MTX, and etanercept as the components of a combined therapeutic set of drugs. Prednisolone was given at 0.5 mg/kg/day (maximum 60 mg) tapered to 0 by 17 weeks. This 6-month trial conducted with 85 children could not show any statistically significant advantage of the combined therapy over MTX monotherapy in achieving clinically inactive disease at 6 months (primary endpoint) or clinical remission at 12 months (secondary endpoint). However, the proportion of responders was higher in the combined-therapy arm.

Finally, single or multiple articular corticosteroid injections may be useful for controlling joint inflammation, inducing disease remission, or as a bridge procedure until systemic immunomodulatory therapy (MTX or biologics) becomes effective [37, 38, 43, 44]. Alternatively, intra-articular corticosteroid therapy may be used to treat arthritis flares in children already receiving such agents [45].

Oligoarticular JIA

Oligoarthritis is the JIA category where intra-articular steroids are the mainstay of treatment. In patients with oligoarticular JIA refractory to NSAIDs, intra-articular corticosteroid therapy is the treatment of choice. However, some pediatric rheumatologists actually use the intra-articular therapy at disease onset to reduce disability and avoid systemic treatment [39, 45]. Intra-articular corticosteroids have been used particularly in children with arthritis that proves refractory to NSAIDs, but they may be used early in the disease to resolve synovitis and to facilitate physiotherapy, the prevention of leg-length discrepancy, and a quicker correction of joints contractures [46, 47].

Table 2 Systemic corticosteroids in systemic JIA

JIA category	Drug	Dose	Patients (*N*)	Concomitant drugs	Study design	Level of evidence[a]	Reference
	M-prednisolone	30 mg/kg /day (max. 1 g)	18	MTX and cyclophosphamide	Open control	4	[31]
	M-prednisolone prednisone	5 mg/kg /day (minipulses) 1 mg/kg/day	22		Cases series	4	[14]
	M-prednisolone	30 mg/kg /day (max. 1 g)	4	MTX and cyclophosphamide	Open control	5	[32]
	M-prednisolone	30 mg/kg /day (max. 1 g)	18	MTX and biologics	Observational	5	[27]
	Prednisone			MTX and biologics	Expert opinion	5	[34]
	Prednisone M-prednisolone	1 mg/kg/day 30 mg/kg/day (max. 1 g)		MTX, anakinra tocilizumab	Expert opinion	5	[25]
	Prednisone			MTX and biologics	Expert opinion	5	[35]

[a]CEBM: http://www.cebm.net/oxford-centre-evidence-based-medicine-levels-evidence-march-2009/

However, some of these patients will eventually need concomitant MTX therapy if remission is not achieved [45]. Four randomized controlled trials comparing different types of steroids showed the higher beneficial effect of triamcinolone hexacetonide over other agents (such as triamcinolone acetonide, methylprednisolone acetate, or betamethasone) [43, 44, 48, 49]. Other observational retrospective studies reported the effectiveness of intra-articular triamcinolone both as hexacetonide or acetonide in patients with oligoarthritis [37, 38, 49, 50].

The only indication for systemic corticosteroid therapy in this group is refractory JIA-related uveitis (see section "Corticosteroids in JIA-related uveitis").

Juvenile Psoriatic Arthritis

For patients with psoriatic arthritis refractory to NSAIDs, intra-articular corticosteroid therapy may be beneficial [38, 39]. The only indication for systemic corticosteroid therapy in this group is refractory JIA-related uveitis (see section "Corticosteroids in JIA-related uveitis").

Enthesitis-Related Arthritis

Patients with ERA are usually treated with NSAIDs and biologics. Additionally, some patients may benefit from intra-articular corticosteroid therapy [38, 39, 51]. Subtalar arthritis, a common inflammation site in ERA, may also be responsive to such treatment [52]. The only indication for systemic corticosteroid therapy in this group is refractory JIA-related uveitis. However, there are some reports in the literature of the successful use of pulse steroid therapy in patients with juvenile spondyloarthropathy [53].

Corticosteroids in MAS

MAS is a severe and potentially fatal clinical condition caused by the excessive activation and proliferation of T lymphocytes and macrophages that lead to a hypercytokinemic state [54]. The resulting clinical syndrome includes fever, cytopenia, lymphadenopathy, hepatosplenomegaly, coagulopathy, and neurological involvement. It is considered a form of secondary hemophagocytic lymphohistiocytosis occurring in a patient with a rheumatic condition. It has been described in patients with systemic JIA and other forms of JIA [55–58]. It probably occurs in 10–15 % of patients with systemic JIA with a mortality rate between 8 and 22 % [58].

Treatment of MAS as part of systemic JIA has developed from anecdotal experience. It has long been based on high-dose corticosteroids, and this therapy – usually in combination with cyclosporine – is still the recommended one today [54–58]. Systemic corticosteroids are usually administered intravenously in the form of pulses (methylprednisolone 30 mg/kg per day for 3 consecutive days) followed by daily methylprednisolone or prednisone 2 mg/kg [33]. There have been reports of patients who respond to oral high-dose corticosteroids [59].

The ACR recommendations for the treatment of JIA devote a separate paragraph for patients with systemic JIA and features suggestive of MAS. Besides the use of anakinra or a calcineurin inhibitor, systemic corticosteroid monotherapy (administered by either oral or intravenous route) was recommended as a separate, initial therapeutic option (level C) [35]. The continuation of corticosteroid monotherapy for more than 2 weeks in patients with continued features of MAS was considered to be inappropriate (level D).

Corticosteroids in JIA-Related Uveitis

Uveitis is an immunologically mediated, severe complication of children with rheumatic diseases, especially JIA [1]. Chronic uveitis may occur in up to 10 % of patients in all JIA categories. It is the most common ocular complication of oligoarticular JIA (affecting up to 30 % of patients), while acute anterior uveitis is characteristic of the spondyloarthropathies or ERA. However, chronic uveitis may also occur in patients with polyarthritis and psoriatic arthritis [60]. Chronic uveitis occurs most frequently in young girls with oligoarthritis and antinuclear antibody (ANA) positivity.

The efficacy and safety of corticosteroids in JIA-related uveitis are not supported by a high evidence level. Moreover, the ACR recommendations for the treatment of JIA have not included guidelines on the treatment of uveitis. The initial therapeutic approach for uveitis includes corticosteroid eye drops and ointment (dexamethasone or methylprednisolone), and mydriatics. Eventually night corticosteroid ointment may be added. Many ophthalmologists use systemic corticosteroids in refractory cases (prednisone 1–2 mg/kg/day orally) to achieve rapid control of inflammation. Intravenous corticosteroids (methylprednisolone, at 30 mg/kg for 3 consecutive days or every other day three times a week) followed by oral corticosteroids (prednisone 0.5–1 mg/kg/day) may be useful in patients with resistant uveitis, optic nerve involvement, serpiginous choroiditis, or panuveitis [61]. Also, subtenon injections of corticosteroids may be required. However, long-term ophthalmic or systemic administration of corticosteroids is frequently ineffective in controlling the disease and may lead to the development of ophthalmic (cataracts and glaucoma) and systemic (Cushing's syndrome) side effects. For these reasons, prolonged systemic corticosteroid therapy should be avoided, and short courses of corticosteroids should be used in acute attacks [62, 63]. Methotrexate and new biologic agents (such as the tumor necrosis factor blockers infliximab and adalimumab) have shown promising results in the treatment of refractory JIA-related uveitis [64–68].

Recently, the German Ophthalmological Society, the Society for Childhood and Adolescent Rheumatology, and the German Society for Rheumatology reached consensus on a standardized treatment strategy for uveitis associated with JIA [69]. According to disease severity, different progressive strategies were defined. After the initial treatment phase with topical steroids (kept at the lowest possible dosage), systemic corticosteroid therapy for a limited period of a few weeks in addition to topical therapy (IIIA) was recommended in refractory patients with severe active uveitis presenting with prognostic factors indicating uveitis-related impending loss of vision (poor vision at initial presentation, hypotony, glaucoma, cataract, macular edema, or dense vitreous body opacification). Additionally, corticosteroid injections to the eye were considered as "rescue therapy" for severe uni- or bilaterally active uveitis associated with prognostic factors indicating uveitis-related impending loss of vision. Systemic immunosuppression was recommended if inactivity cannot be achieved under topical corticosteroid drops and/or within 3 months while under systemic maintenance corticosteroid therapy (prednisolone 0.15 mg/kg/day).

Intra-articular Corticosteroid Therapy in JIA

The earliest report on intra-articular steroids was published in 1951 [70]. During the following decades this treatment approach has been used with remarkable effectiveness, especially in oligoarthritis. Although several preparations are available for injections in children, all of them are not on the market in every country. These preparations are hydrocortisone acetate, methylprednisolone acetate, triamcinolone acetonide, triamcinolone hexacetonide, and betamethasone. They all have different pharmacological properties: The solubility of triamcinolone acetonide and hexacetonide is lower than in other preparations [45].

Intra-articular corticosteroid therapy may be an effective therapy for inflammatory joint disease in all categories of JIA but efficacy may vary according to JIA subtype. It may even lead to long-lasting disease remission, at least in oligoarticular JIA [37]. In a study by Breit et al., duration of improvement was 121 weeks in oligoarthritis, 105 weeks in rheumatoid factor-negative polyarthritis, 63 weeks in rheumatoid factor–positive polyarthritis, 47 weeks in ERA, and 36 weeks in systemic JIA [36]. Lanni et al. retrospectively assessed outcome in patients with JIA who had received single and multiple intra-articular triamcinolone hexacetonide injections. The cumulative probability of survival without flare for patients injected in one, two, or three or more joints was 70, 45, and 44 %, respectively, at 1 year; 61, 32, and 30 %, respectively, at 2 years; and 37, 22, and 19 %, respectively, at 3 years. Patients with systemic JIA carried a greater risk of flare than patients with other JIA diagnoses [39].

Triamcinolone hexacetonide is the drug of choice because of its high efficacy and long-lasting effect. Controlled studies have demonstrated the superiority of intra-articular triamcinolone hexacetonide over triamcinolone acetonide in the treatment of JIA, likely due to its longer duration of action [44, 71]. Zulian et al. demonstrated in two randomized double-blinded trials that triamcinolone hexacetonide was more effective than triamcinolone acetonide, even when this drug was used at higher doses (2 mg/kg, maximum 80 mg) [43, 44]. However, for smaller joints or joints that are not easy to assess, the use of more soluble corticosteroids – such as methylprednisone – is advised [72]. Children who receive triamcinolone hexacetonide benefit from a significantly longer period of remission, and the effect of triamcinolone acetonide is longer than the one of methylprednisone, making it preferable for joint injections [48, 73]. The conventional dose of triamcinolone hexacetonide is 1 mg/kg per large joint [45], but needs to be adjusted also according to the joint space size (i.e., not injecting against pressure to avoid leakage). Some children have received higher doses of triamcinolone hexacetonide (2 mg/kg per large joint) without overt problems [74]. An age–weight–joint-based corticosteroid dose protocol was developed by Young et al. [75] using from 1 to 20 mg in each injection, the higher dose being for larger joints in older and heavier patients. In difficult-to-access joints, fluoroscopically or ultrasound-guided injections can be administered [52].

The intra-articular injection of triamcinolone hexacetonide is a safe procedure [37, 76–78]. Few side effects occur in less than 5 % of injected patients. Subcutaneous tissue atrophy (transient or persistent), skin hypopigmentation, periarticular or joint capsule calcification, erythema and pain, and pruritus have been reported in the literature [45, 52, 75]. Local postinjection inflammatory features might be related to steroid crystal-induced synovitis [79]. A potentially more severe adverse event is the femoral head necrosis reported in injected hips [80]. Iatrogenic transient Cushing's syndrome in children who received intra-articular injections with triamcinolone acetonide has also been rarely reported [73]. Symptoms of Cushing's syndrome occurred as early as 2 weeks after the injections in patients who had received from one to several joint injections with a total triamcinolone acetonide dose ranging between 11.7 and 14.5 mg/kg.

Corticosteroid injection may be a useful procedure for the prevention and treatment of morbidities associated with temporomandibular joint (TMJ) arthritis in JIA. In the last few years, iontophoresis has been proposed as a novel, effective, and safe strategy for corticosteroid delivery into the joints, specifically for TMJs [81]. Although the TMJ is typically involved in polyarticular and oligoarticular JIA, it is a fairly common site of inflammation in all types of JIA [82].

A summary of different studies on the use of intra-articular corticosteroid therapy in JIA is given in Table 3.

Conclusions

The efficacy of corticosteroid therapy has been demonstrated in patients with JIA. Several drawbacks have limited the validity of different reports and studies (mostly retrospective) on systemic therapy that support their use in clinical practice: lack of validated outcome measures, lack of randomized controlled trials, the frequent use of concomitant therapies, heterogeneity in the treatment subjects, and small sample size. Different approaches for the treatment of the various types of JIA include corticosteroids, whether systemically or locally applied. The most frequent and important indications are the presence of extra-articular features such as refractory anemia, carditis, serositis, or MAS. The use of low-dose corticosteroid as a bridging strategy may prove advantageous in polyarthritis. In the past few years, recommendations for the treatment of JIA elaborated by scientific organizations have aided us to standardize the use of systemic agents in different clinical scenarios and to reduce or avoid the use of ineffective plans that include long-term systemic corticosteroids. On the other hand, intra-articular steroids (triamcinolone hexacetonide) have proven highly efficacious and safe in well-designed trials, particularly in patients with oligoarticular JIA. Well-designed trials may provide a stronger evidence level for the recommendation of the use of corticosteroids in JIA.

Table 3 Intra-articular corticosteroid therapy in JIA

JIA category	Drug	Dose	Patients (*N*)	Concomitant drugs	Study design	Level of evidence[a]	Reference
Systemic	Triamcinolone hexacetonide	10–40 mg	13	Yes	Observational retrospective	4	[37]
Systemic	Triamcinolone hexacetonide		194 JIA Systemic?	?	Observational retrospective	4	[36]
Systemic	Triamcinolone acetonide	0.5–1 mg	2	Yes (DMARDs and biologics)	Observational retrospective	4	[38]
Systemic	Triamcinolone acetonide	1 mg/kg (max 20–40 mg)	20	Yes (DMARDs and biologics)	Observational retrospective	4	[39]
Systemic	Triamcinolone hexacetonide (large joints) Methylprednisolone acetate (small and difficult-to-access joints)			?	Observational retrospective	4	[40]
Oligoarticular	Triamcinolone hexacetonide betamethasone		23	Yes	Randomized Double-blind	3b	[49]
Oligoarticular	Triamcinolone hexacetonide Methylprednisolone acetate	0.5 mg/kg 1.5 mg/kg	40	Yes	Randomized Blinded	3b	[48]
Oligoarticular	Triamcinolone hexacetonide	10–40 mg	43	Yes	Observational retrospective	4	[37]
Oligoarticular	Triamcinolone hexacetonide Triamcinolone acetonide	1 mg/kg 1 mg/kg (max. 40 mg)	85	Yes	Randomized Blinded	3b	[43]
Oligoarticular	Triamcinolone hexacetonide Triamcinolone acetonide		48	Yes	Observational retrospective	4	[71]

Oligoarticular	Triamcinolone hexacetonide Triamcinolone acetonide	1 mg/kg (max. 40 mg) 2 mg/kg (max. 80 mg)	37	Yes	Randomized Double-Blind	3b	[44]
Oligoarticular	Triamcinolone acetonide	0.5–1 mg	17	Yes	Observational retrospective	4	[38]
Oligoarticular	Triamcinolone acetonide	0.5–1 mg	12	Yes	Observational retrospective	4	[50]
Oligoarticular	Triamcinolone hexacetonide	1 mg/kg (max. 40 mg)	171	Yes	Observational retrospective	4	[39]
Polyarticular	Triamcinolone hexacetonide	10–40 mg	5	Yes	Observational retrospective	4	[37]
Polyarticular	Triamcinolone hexacetonide Triamcinolone acetonide	1 mg/kg (max. 40 mg) 2 mg/kg (max. 80 mg)	5	Yes	Randomized Double-Blind	3b	[44]
Polyarticular	Triamcinolone acetonide	0.5–1 mg	4	Yes	Observational retrospective	4	[38]
Polyarticular	Triamcinolone hexacetonide	1 mg/kg (max. 40 mg)	70	Yes	Observational retrospective	4	[39]
Psoriatic	Triamcinolone acetonide	0.5–1 mg	4	Yes	Observational retrospective	4	[38]
Psoriatic	Triamcinolone hexacetonide	1 mg/kg (max. 40 mg)	9	Yes	Observational retrospective	4	[39]
Enthesitis-related	Triamcinolone hexacetonide		13	Yes	Observational	4	[51]
Enthesitis-related	Triamcinolone acetonide	0.5–1 mg	10	Yes	Observational retrospective	4	[38]

(continued)

Table 3 (continued)

JIA category	Drug	Dose	Patients (N)	Concomitant drugs	Study design	Level of evidence[a]	Reference
Enthesitis-related	Triamcinolone hexacetonide	1 mg/kg (max. 40 mg)	8	Yes	Observational retrospective	4	[39]
Undifferentiated	Triamcinolone hexacetonide	1 mg/kg (max. 40 mg)	8	Yes	Observational retrospective	4	[39]

[a]CEBM: www.cebm.net/levelsofevidence.asp

References

1. Petty RE, Cassidy JT (2011) Chronic arthritis in childhood. In: Cassidy JT, Petty RE, Laxer RM, Lindsley CB (eds) Textbook of pediatric rheumatology, 6th edn. Elsevier Saunders, Philadelphia, pp 211–235
2. Prakken B, Albani S, Martini A (2011) Juvenile idiopathic arthritis. Lancet 377:2138–2149
3. Petty RE, Southwood TR, Manners P et al (2004) International League of Associations for Rheumatology classification of juvenile idiopathic arthritis: second revision, Edmonton, 2001. J Rheumatol 31:390–392
4. Ansell BM, Bywaters EGL (1957) Growth in Still's disease. Ann Rheum Dis 15:295–319
5. De Benedetti F, Brunner HI, Ruperto N et al (2012) Randomized trial of tocilizumab in systemic juvenile idiopathic arthritis. N Engl J Med 367:2385–2395
6. Ruperto N, Brunner HI, Quartier P et al (2012) Two randomized trials of canakinumab in systemic juvenile idiopathic arthritis. N Engl J Med 367:2396–2406
7. Quartier P, Allantaz F, Cimaz R et al (2011) A multicentre, randomised, double-blind, placebo-controlled trial with the interleukin-1 receptor antagonist anakinra in patients with systemic-onset juvenile idiopathic arthritis (ANAJIS trial). Ann Rheum Dis 70:747–754
8. Vastert SJ, de Jager W, Noordman BJ et al (2014) Effectiveness of first-line treatment with recombinant interleukin-1 receptor antagonist in steroid-naive patients with new-onset systemic juvenile idiopathic arthritis: results of a prospective cohort study. Arthritis Rheumatol 66:1034–1043
9. Ilowite NT, Prather K, Lokhnygina Y et al (2014) The randomized placebo phase study of rilonacept in the treatment of systemic juvenile idiopathic arthritis (RAPPORT). Arthritis Rheum. doi:10.1002/art.38699
10. Morand E, Goulding J (1993) Glucocorticoids in rheumatoid arthritis –mediators and mechanisms. Br J Rheumatol 32:816–819
11. Loftus J, Allen R, Hesp R et al (1991) Randomized, double-blind trial of deflazacort versus prednisone in juvenile chronic (rheumatoid) arthritis: a relatively bone-sparing effect of deflazacort. Pediatrics 88:428–436
12. Loftus JK, Reeve J, Hesp R et al (1993) Deflazacort in juvenile arthritis. J Rheumatol Suppl 37:40–42
13. Beukelman T, Ringold S, Davis TE et al (2012) Disease modifying anti-rheumatic drug use in the treatment of juvenile idiopathic arthritis: a cross-sectional analysis of the CARRA registry. J Rheumatol 39:1867–1874
14. Picco P, Gattorno M, Buoncompagni A et al (1996) 6-methylprednisolone "mini-pulses": a new modality of glucocorticoid treatment in systemic onset juvenile chronic arthritis. Scand J Rheumatol 25:24–27
15. Miller JJ (1980) Prolonged use of large intravenous steroid pulses in the rheumatic diseases of children. Pediatrics 65:989–994
16. Kotianiemi A, Savolainen A, Kautiainen H et al (1993) Estimation of central osteopenia in children with chronic polyarthritis treated with glucocorticoids. Pediatrics 91:1127–1130
17. Markula-Patjas KP, Valta HL, Kerttula LI et al (2012) Prevalence of vertebral compression fractures and associated factors in children and adolescents with severe juvenile idiopathic arthritis. J Rheumatol 39:365–373
18. Valta H, Lahdenne V, Jalonko P et al (2007) Bone health and growth in glucocorticoid-treated patients with juvenile idiopathic arthritis. J Rheumatol 34:831–836
19. Wang SJ, Yang YH, Lin YT et al (2002) Attained adult height in juvenile rheumatoid arthritis with or without corticosteroid treatment. Clin Rheumatol 21:363–368
20. Simon D, Fernando C, Czernichow P et al (2002) Linear growth and final height in patients with systemic juvenile idiopathic arthritis treated with longterm glucocorticoids. J Rheumatol 29:1296–1300
21. Byron MA, Jackson J, Ansell BM (1983) Effect of different corticosteroid regimes on hypothalamic-pituitary-adrenal axis and growth in juvenile chronic arthritis. J R Soc Med 76:452–457

22. Souza L, Machado SH, Bredemeier M et al (2006) Effect of inflammatory activity and glucorticoid use on nutritional variables in patients with juvenile idiopathic arthritis. J Rheumatol 33:601–608
23. Shiff NJ, Brant R, Guzman J et al (2013) Glucocorticoid-related changes in body mass index among children and adolescents with rheumatic diseases. Arthritis Care Res 65:113–121
24. Hugle B, Hass JP, Benseler S (2013) Treatment preferences in juvenile idiopathic arthritis- a comparative analysis in two health care systems. Pediatr Rheumatol Online J 11:3
25. Dewitt ES, Kimura Y, Beukelman T et al (2012) Consensus treatment plans for new-onset systemic juvenile idiopathic arthritis. Arthritis Care Res 64:1001–1010
26. Otten MH, Anink J, Prince FHM et al (2014) Trends in prescription of biological agents and outcomes of juvenile idiopathic arthritis: results of the Dutch national Arthritis and Biologics in Children Register. Ann Rheum Dis. doi:10.1136/annrheumdis-2013-204641
27. Adebajo AO, Hall MA (1998) The use of intravenous pulsed methylprednisolone in the treatment of systemic-onset juvenile chronic arthritis. J Rheumatol 37:1240–1242
28. Ravelli A, Lattanzi B, Consolaro A et al (2011) Glucocorticoids in paediatric rheumatology. Clin Exp Rheumatol 29:148–152
29. Wallace CA (2006) Current management of juvenile idiopathic arthritis. Best Pract Res Clin Rheumatol 20:279–300
30. Klein-Gitelman MS, Pachman LM (1998) Intravenous corticosteroids: adverse reactions are more variable than expected in children. J Rheumatol 25:1995–2002
31. Shaikov AV, Maximov AA, Speransky AI et al (1992) Repetitive use of pulse therapy with methylprednisolone and cyclophosphamide in addition to oral methotrexate in children with systemic juvenile rheumatoid arthritis–preliminary results of a longterm study. J Rheumatol 19:612–616
32. Wallace CA, Sherry DD (1997) Trial of intravenous pulse cyclophosphamide and methylprednisolone in the treatment of severe systemic-onset juvenile rheumatoid arthritis. Arthritis Rheum 40:1852–1855
33. Ilowite NT, Sandborg CI, Feldman BM et al (2012) Algorithm development for corticosteroid management in systemic juvenile idiopathic arthritis trial using consensus methodology. Pediatr Rheumatol Online J 10:31. doi:10.1186/1546-0096-10-31
34. Beukelman T, Patkar NM, Saag KG et al (2011) 2011 American College of Rheumatology recommendations for the treatment of juvenile idiopathic arthritis: initiation and safety monitoring of therapeutic agents for the treatment of arthritis and systemic features. Arthritis Care Res 63:465–482
35. Ringold S, Weiss PF, Beukelman T et al (2013) 2013 Update of the 2011 American College of Rheumatology recommendations for the treatment of juvenile idiopathic arthritis: recommendations for the medical therapy of children with systemic juvenile idiopathic arthritis and tuberculosis screening among children receiving biological medications. Arthritis Care Res 65:1551–1563
36. Breit W, Frosch M, Meyer U et al (2000) A sub-group specific evaluation of the efficacy of intra-articular triamcinolone hexacetonide in juvenile chronic arthritis. J Rheumatol 27:2696–2702
37. Padeh S, Passwell J (1998) Intraarticular corticosteroid injection in the management of children with chronic arthritis. Arthritis Rheum 41:1210–1214
38. Ünsal E, Makay B (2008) Intra-articular triamcinolone in juvenile idiopathic arthritis. Indian Pediatr 45:995–997
39. Lanni S, Bertamino M, Consolaro A et al (2011) Outcome and predicting factors of single and multiple intra-articular corticosteroid injections in children with juvenile idiopathic arthritis. Rheumatology 50:1627–1634
40. Papadopoulou C, Kostik M, Gonzalez-Fernandez MI et al (2013) Delineating the role of multiple intraarticular corticosteroid injections in the management of juvenile idiopathic arthritis in the biologic era. Arthritis Care Res 65:1112–1120
41. Ilowite NT, Laxer RM (2011) Pharmacology and drug therapy. In: Cassidy J, Petty R, Laxer RM et al (eds) Textbook of pediatric rheumatology, 6th edn. Saunders, Philadelphia, pp 71–126

42. Wallace CA, Giannini EH, Spalding SJ et al (2012) Trial of aggressive therapy in polyarticular juvenile idiopathic arthritis. Arthritis Rheum 64:2012–2021
43. Zulian F, Martini G, Gobber D et al (2003) Comparison of intra-articular triamcinolone hexacetonide and triamcinolone acetonide in oligoarticular juvenile idiopathic arthritis. Rheumatology 42:1254–1259
44. Zulian F, Martini G, Gobber D et al (2004) Triamcinolone acetonide and hexacetonide intra-articular treatment of symmetrical joints in juvenile idiopathic arthritis: a double-blind trial. Rheumatology 43:1288–1291
45. Cleary AG, Murphy HD, Davidson JE (2003) Intra-articular corticosteroid injections in juvenile idiopathic arthritis. Arch Dis Child 88:192–196
46. Allen R, Gross K, Laxer R et al (1986) Intraarticular triamcinolone hexacetonide in the management of chronic arthritis in children. Arthritis Rheum 29:997–1001
47. Sherry D, Stein L, Reed A (1999) Prevention of leg length discrepancy in young children with pauciarticular juvenile rheumatoid arthritis by treatment with intraraticular steroids. Arthritis Rheum 42:2330–2333
48. Honkanen V, Rautonen J, Pelkonen P (1993) Intra-articular glucocorticoids in early juvenile chronic arthritis. Acta Paediatr 82:1072–1074
49. Balogh Z, Ruzsonyi E (1987) Triamcinolone hexacetonide versus betamethasone. A double – blind comparative study of the long-term effects of intra-articular steroids in patients with juvenile chronic arthritis. Scand J Rheumatol 67:80–82
50. Verma S, Gupta R, Lodha R et al (2009) Feasibility and efficacy of intraarticular steroids in juvenile idiopathic arthritis (JIA). Indian Pediatr 46:264–265
51. Job-Deslandre C, Menkes CJ (1990) Complications of intraarticular injections of triamcinolone hexacetonide in chronic arthritis in children. Clin Exp Rheumatol 8:413–416
52. Cahill AM, Cho SS, Baskin KM et al (2007) Benefit of fluoroscopically guided intraarticular, long-acting corticosteroid injection for subtalar arthritis in juvenile idiopathic arthritis. Pediatr Radiol 37:544–548
53. Job-Deslandre C, Menkes CJ (1991) Administration of methylprednisolone pulse in chronic arthritis in children. Clin Exp Rheumatol 9(Suppl 6):15–18
54. Ravelli A, Grom AA, Behrens EM et al (2012) Macrophage activation syndrome as part of systemic juvenile idiopathic arthritis: diagnosis, genetics, pathophysiology and treatment. Genes Immun 13:289–2989
55. Stéphan JL, Koné-Paut I, Galambrun C et al (2001) Reactive haemophagocytic syndrome in children with inflammatory disorders. A retrospective study of 24 patients. Rheumatology 40:1285–1292
56. Hadchouel M, Prieur AM, Griscelli S (1985) Acute hemorrhagic, hepatic, and neurologic manifestations in juvenile rheumatoid arthritis: possible relationship to drugs or infection. J Pediatr 106:561–566
57. Stéphan JL, Zeller J, Hubert P et al (1993) Macrophage activation syndrome and rheumatic disease in childhood: a report of four new cases. Clin Exp Rheumatol 11:451–456
58. Sawhney S, Woo P, Murray KJ (2001) Macrophage activation syndrome: a potentially fatal complication of rheumatic disorders. Arch Dis Child 85:421–426
59. Cuende E, Vesga JC, Pérez LB et al (2011) Macrophage activation syndrome as the initial manifestation of systemic onset juvenile idiopathic arthritis. Clin Exp Rheumatol 19:764–765
60. Moretti D, Cianchi I, Vanucci G et al (2013) Psoriatic juvenile idiopathic arthritis associated with uveitis: a case report. Case Rep Rheumatol 2013:595890
61. Simonini G, Cantarini L, Bresci C et al (2010) Current approaches to autoinmune chronic uveitis in children. Autoimmun Rev 9:674–683
62. Anesi SD, Foster CS (2012) Importance of recognizing and preventing blindness from juvenile idiopathic arthritis-associated uveitis. Arthritis Care Res 64:653–657
63. Nguyen QD, Foster CS (1998) Saving the vision of children with juvenile rheumatoid arthritis-associated uveitis. JAMA 280:1133–1134
64. Reiff A, Takei S, Sadeghi S et al (2001) Etanercept therapy in children with treatment-resistant uveitis. Arthritis Rheum 44:1411–1415

65. Rajaraman RT, Kimura Y, Li S et al (2006) Retrospective case review of pediatric patients with uveitis treated with infliximab. Ophthalmology 113:308–314
66. Saurenmann RK, Levin AV, Rose JB et al (2006) Tumour necrosis factor alpha inhibitors in the treatment of childhood uveitis. Rheumatology 45:982–989
67. Zannin ME, Birolo C, Gerloni VM et al (2013) Safety and efficacy of infliximab and adalimumab for refractory uveitis in juvenile idiopathic arthritis: 1-year followup data from the Italian Registry. J Rheumatol 40:74–79
68. Simonini G, Taddio A, Cattalini M et al (2011) Prevention of flare recurrences in childhood-refractory chronic uveitis: an open-label comparative study of adalimumab versus infliximab. Arthritis Care Res 63:612–618
69. Heiligenhaus A, Michel H, Schumacher C et al (2012) Evidence-based, interdisciplinary guidelines for anti-inflammatory treatment of uveitis associated with juvenile idiopathic arthritis. Rheumatol Int 32:1121–1133
70. Hollander J, Brown E, Jessar R et al (1951) Hydrocortisone and cortisone injected into arthritis joints: comparative effects of and use of hydrocortisone as a local anesthetic agents. JAMA 147:1629–1635
71. Eberhard BA, Sison MC, Gottlieb BS et al (2004) Comparison of the intraarticular effectiveness of triamcinolone hexacetonide and triamcinolone acetonide in treatment juvenile rheumatoid arthritis. J Rheumatol 31:2507–2512
72. Scott C, Meirin S, Filocamo G et al (2010) A reappraisal of intra-articular corticosteroid therapy in juvenile idiopathic arthritis. Clin Exp Rheumatol 5:774–781
73. Bloom BJ, Alario AJ, Miller LC (2011) Intra-articular corticosteroid therapy for juvenile idiopathic arthritis: report of an experiential cohort and literature review. Rheumatol Int 31:749–756
74. Alsufyani K, Ortiz-Alvarez O, Cabral DA et al (2004) Relative ineffectiveness of triamcinolone acetonide in the treatment of juvenile idiopathic arthritis. Arthritis Rheum 11:3733–3740
75. Young CM, Shiels WE, Coley BD et al (2012) Ultrasound-guided corticosteroid injection therapy for juvenile idiopathic arthritis: 12-year care experience. Pediatr Radiol 42:1481–1489
76. Sparling M, Malleson P, Wood B et al (1990) Radiographic followup of joints injected with triamcinolone hexacetonide for the management of childhood arthritis. Arthritis Rheum 33:821–826
77. Huppertz H-I, Tschammler A, Horwitz AE et al (1995) Intraarticular corticosteroids for chronic arthritis in children: efficacy and effects on cartilage and growth. J Pediatr 127:317–321
78. Eich GF, Halle F, Hodler J et al (1994) Juvenile chronic arthritis: imaging of the knees and hips before and after intraarticular steroid injection. Pediatr Radiol 24:558–563
79. Hertzberger-ten Cate R, de Vries-van der Vlugt BCM, van Suijlekom-Smit LWA et al (1991) Intra-articular steroids in pauciarticular juvenile chronic arthritis, type 1. Eur J Pediatr 150:170–172
80. Neidel J, Boehnke M, Küster RM (2002) The efficacy and safety of intraarticular corticosteroid therapy for coxitis in juvenile rheumatoid arthritis. Arthritis Rheum 46:1620–1628
81. Mina R, Melson P, Powell S et al (2011) Effectiveness of dexamethasone iontophoresis for temporomandibular joint involvement in juvenile idiopathic arthritis. Arthritis Care Res 63:1511–1516
82. Billiau AD, Hu Y, Verdonck A et al (2007) Temporomandibular joint arthritis in juvenile idiopathic arthritis: prevalence, clinical and radiological signs, and relation to dentofacial morphology. J Rheumatol 34:1925–1933

Systemic Corticosteroids in Childhood Vasculitides

Gašper Markelj and Tadej Avčin

Introduction

Owing to the complexity and multisystemic nature of the disease, children with vasculitis often present to different pediatric subspecialists such as rheumatologists, cardiologists, nephrologists, and dermatologists. Different types of inflammatory infiltrate that may be predominantly neutrophilic, eosinophilic, or mononuclear affect the blood vessel wall. Classification of the most common childhood vasculitides was recently revised and is based on predominant vessel size and the presence of granulomatous vasculitis (Table 1) [1].

Clinical presentation of the most common childhood vasculitides usually develops abruptly, and diagnostic characteristics become apparent in a few days. In some less common vasculitides, various signs and symptoms may develop over weeks or months. Establishing the diagnosis of vasculitis requires a high index of suspicion and is often difficult and delayed. Clinical features such as fever, weight loss, fatigue of unknown origin, various skin lesions (palpable purpura, vasculitic urticaria, livedo reticularis, nodules, ulcers), neurological manifestations (headache, focal neurological signs), pain or inflammation of joints and muscles, serositis, hypertension, pulmonary infiltrates or hemorrhage together with laboratory features of increased inflammatory markers [erythrocyte sedimentation rate, C-reactive protein (CRP), leukocytosis], anemia, eosinophilia, hematuria, elevated factor VIII–related antigen (von Willebrand factor), presence of antineutrophil cytoplasmic antibodies (ANCA), circulating immune complexes, and cryoglobulins suggest a possible diagnosis. A definitive diagnosis often requires additional vessel imaging, such as magnetic resonance angiography or conventional angiography, and frequently biopsy of one or more sites.

G. Markelj • T. Avčin (✉)
Department of Allergology, Rheumatology and Clinical Immunology, University Children's Hospital, University Medical Center Ljubljana, Ljubljana, Slovenia
e-mail: tadej.avcin@kclj.si

R. Cimaz (ed.), *Systemic Corticosteroids for Inflammatory Disorders in Pediatrics*, DOI 10.1007/978-3-319-16056-6_7

Table 1 EULAR/PReS classification of childhood vasculitis [1]

I. Predominantly large vessel vasculitis	Takayasu arteritis
II. Predominantly medium-sized vessel vasculitis	Kawasaki disease
	Childhood polyarteritis nodosa
	Cutaneous polyarteritis
III. Predominantly small vessel vasculitis	
A. Granulomatous	Granulomatosis with polyangiitis (GPA), formerly known as Wegener's granulomatosis
	Churg–Strauss syndrome
B. Nongranulomatous	Microscopic polyangiitis
	Henoch–Schönlein purpura
	Isolated cutaneous leukocytoclastic vasculitis
	Hypocomplementemic urticarial vasculitis
IV. Other vasculitides	Behçet's disease
	Vasculitis secondary to infection (including hepatitis B-associated polyarteritis nodosa), malignancies, and drugs (including hypersensitivity vasculitis)
	Vasculitis associated with systemic connective tissue diseases
	Isolated vasculitis of the central nervous system
	Cogan syndrome
	Unclassified

Besides difficulties in establishing a diagnosis, assessment of vasculitic disease activity is often challenging and the outcome of some vasculitides may be serious or fatal [2–4]. Various forms of vasculitis account for 1–6 % of pediatric rheumatic diseases, but the true incidence and prevalence are unknown. The two most common childhood vasculitides, accounting for 60–80 % of all types of vasculitis, are Henoch–Schönlein purpura (HSP) and Kawasaki disease (KD). All other forms of vasculitis are uncommon – Takayasu arteritis (TA), polyarteritis nodosa (PAN) – or rare – granulomatosis with polyangiitis (GPA), central nervous system (CNS) vasculitis. There are, however, large geographical differences in relative disease frequency, with KD and TA being more prevalent in Japan and PAN more common in Turkey [2, 4, 5]. Several aspects of corticosteroid therapy in the most common childhood vasculitides are presented in this chapter.

Henoch–Schönlein Purpura

HSP is the most common childhood vasculitis. It is a systemic vasculitis with multiorgan involvement and presents with palpable purpura, arthritis or arthralgia, abdominal pain, with the possible addition of gastrointestinal hemorrhage and renal disease. The presence of purpura is a compulsory criterion for the diagnosis, other signs or symptoms are present more variably. Other organs can also be involved including central nervous system vasculitis with seizures, coma, hemorrhage, Guillain–Barré syndrome, central and peripheral neuropathy, as well as involvement of the respiratory system with recurrent epistaxis, pulmonary hemorrhages, interstitial pneumonitis, parotitis, carditis, and stenosing urethritis. In boys the most frequent additional manifestation is scrotal pain and swelling [6–8].

The reported incidence of HSP varies between 10 and 30 cases per 100,000 children with an equal incidence in male and female patients. Most cases present in children younger than 10 years of age with mean age of presentation at 6 years. It occurs predominantly in the cold months of the year, often preceded by an upper respiratory tract infection. This suggests a potential infectious trigger and multiple case reports describe an association with various respiratory pathogens, most commonly with streptococcus, staphylococcus, and parainfluenza [2, 6–8].

The characteristic pathological feature of HSP vasculitis is a deposition of IgA antibodies – containing immune complexes in the vessel walls of the affected organs and kidney mesangium. Abnormal glycosylation of immunoglobulin A1 molecules predispose patients with HSP to form large immune complexes with impaired clearance. They are deposited in small vessel walls of the affected organs and in the kidney mesangium and trigger immune response with inflammatory reaction.

Clinical Manifestations

Cutaneous Involvement

Skin involvement is essential for the diagnosis to be made. The most common manifestations are palpable purpura and petechiae, but other forms of skin involvement like erythematous, macular, urticarial, and bullous rashes have been observed. Skin involvement is usually distributed symmetrically most prominently over the extensor surfaces of the lower limbs, buttocks, and forearms – on pressure-bearing surfaces (Figs. 1 and 2). Changes on the trunk and face are occasionally described in younger children with edema over the dorsa of the hands and feet as well as around the eyes and forehead. In 25–30 % of children with HSP, recurrence of purpura is observed.

Arthritis

Three quarters of children with HSP have arthritis or arthralgia. The most commonly affected joints are the large joints of the lower extremities. There is marked periarticular swelling and tenderness, usually without erythema, warmth, and effusion. The joint disease is transient and resolves within a few days to 1 week without chronic damage.

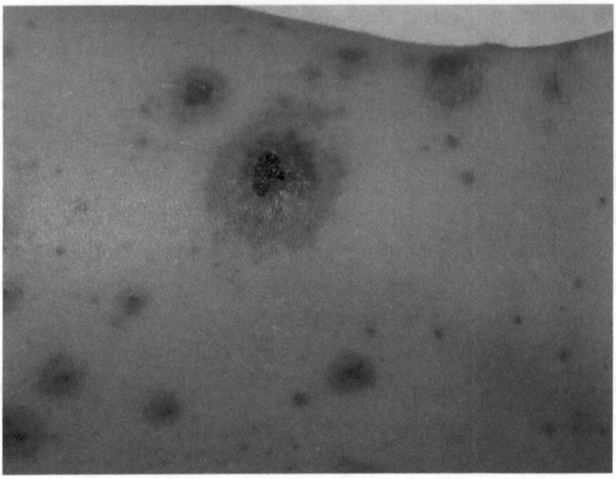

Fig. 1 Hemorrhagic necrotic skin lesions in a patient with Henoch–Schönlein purpura

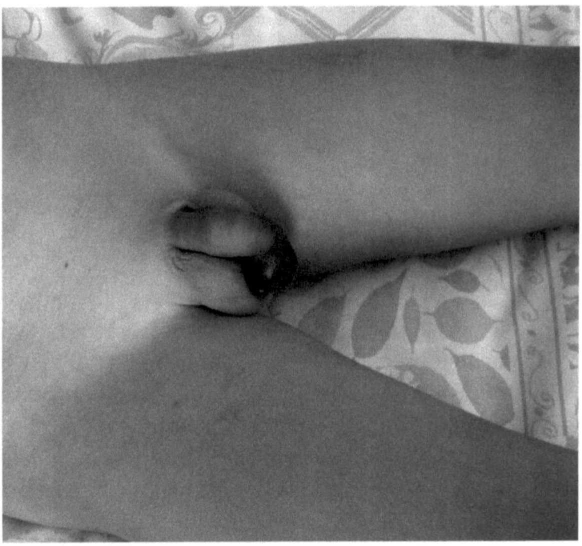

Fig. 2 Penile involvement in a patient with Henoch–Schönlein purpura

Gastrointestinal Manifestations

Edemas and submucosal and intramural hemorrhage due to vasculitis of the bowel wall cause diffuse abdominal pain in approximately two thirds of children with HSP. The proximal small bowel is most commonly affected. Symptoms usually appear within 1 week after onset of the rash, but in up to one third of cases they may precede other manifestations. The most common severe gastrointestinal complication is intussusception, which occurs in 3–4 % of patients. It presents with severe, often colicky abdominal pain and vomiting. Other severe, although less common gastrointestinal complications, include gangrene of the bowel, bowel perforation, massive hemorrhage, acute pancreatitis, enteritis, and hepatobiliary involvement.

Renal Disease

Renal involvement with glomerulonephritis is reported in approximately one third of children with HSP. It usually presents with isolated microscopic hematuria; there might be a variable degree of proteinuria with normal renal function. In less than 10 % of cases it may be a serious, potentially life-threatening complication with acute nephritic syndrome with hypertension and renal failure. It seldom precedes the onset of rash and usually develops within 4 weeks after disease onset. The extent of the disease can be determined in the initial 3 months, and in a few children nephritis can occur much later in the course, sometimes after numerous cutaneous recurrences.

Treatment

The use of glucocorticosteroids (GCs) in HSP has been a source of controversy and debate [9–13]. In the majority of cases, management of HSP includes supportive care with maintenance of good hydration, nutrition, electrolyte balance, and control of pain and hypertension. Although GCs have a dramatic influence on decreasing the severity of joint and cutaneous involvement of the disease they are usually not indicated for management of these manifestations. The evidence of using early GC treatment to shorten duration of abdominal pain and to decrease the risk of intussusception and surgical intervention is based only on case reports and small studies and is not strong enough to recommend it to all patients with HSP and abdominal involvement, since the majority of patients improve spontaneously [14]. GCs are generally used for patients with HSP and severe abdominal pain and hemorrhage, with prompt symptomatic improvement. Ronkainen et al. reported reduced abdominal and joint pain with prednisone of 1 mg/kg/day for 2 weeks, with weaning over the subsequent 2 weeks [15]. However, studies have not demonstrated a clear advantage of prednisolone over supportive therapy.

Short-term GC therapy is effective in the management of pain in severe orchitis. In pulmonary hemorrhage, which is a rare but potentially fatal complication of HSP, aggressive immunosuppressive treatment with a combination of intravenous methylprednisolone pulses and other immunosuppressive agents is used.

A recent Cochrane Review and other long-term studies showed there is no evidence from randomized controlled studies that the use of GCs can prevent kidney disease in children with HSP or change the long-term prognosis of renal involvement [16]. Urine and blood pressure abnormalities 8 years after HSP are associated with nephritis at its onset. However, prednisone can be effective in treating renal symptoms: 61 % of renal symptoms resolve in patients treated with prednisone, compared with 34 % of patients treated with placebo [17]. Mild renal involvement with microscopic hematuria or mild proteinuria does not require immunosuppressive treatment, but these patients need close follow-up. GCs are still the main therapy for rapidly progressive glomerulonephritis or nephrotic syndrome, which is usually accompanied by crescents on kidney biopsy. Although the quality of evidence is low, pulse intravenous methylprednisolone followed by a 3–6-month course of oral steroids with the addition of cyclophosphamide or cyclosporine A is used. Additional treatment in small studies included intravenous immunoglobulins, plasmapheresis, and anti-clotting therapy [5, 9–13, 15, 18, 19].

Prognosis

In two thirds of children, disease is self-limiting with excellent spontaneous resolution of symptoms and signs. HSP recurs spontaneously or with repeated respiratory tract infections in one third of children usually in the first 6 weeks. Recurrent episodes are usually shorter and milder than the preceding one.

In the short term, morbidity and mortality are associated with gastrointestinal tract lesions or central nervous system vasculitis. The long-term morbidity of HSP is related to the degree of HSP nephritis. Overall, less than 5 % of children with HSP progress to end-stage renal failure. Poor prognostic factors are development of a major indication of renal disease within the first 6 months of disease onset, occurrence of numerous exacerbations, renal failure at onset, hypertension, or increased number of glomeruli with crescents on renal biopsy [2, 4, 6–9].

Kawasaki Disease

KD is the second most common vasculitis in childhood. It is an acute self-limiting vasculitis of unknown origin with clinical signs of prolonged fever, polymorphous rash, nonexudative conjunctivitis, mucosal changes, cervical lymphadenopathy, and erythema or desquamation of the extremities. Untreated KD can have severe complications and significant morbidity or even mortality. It can progress in 25 % of cases to cause coronary artery abnormalities, such as dilatation and ectasia; 2–3 % of untreated patients die as a result of coronary vasculitis. KD is a leading cause of acquired cardiovascular disease in children and is potentially an important cause of long-term cardiac disease in adult life. Since adequate and timely therapy can largely prevent these complications, early and accurate diagnosis is of great importance.

The disease has a higher incidence in Asian populations with a male predominance; there is marked seasonality with heightened incidence in winter and early spring in temperate climates. The majority (85 %) of children with KD are younger than 5 years.

The exact mechanisms of the disease are still unresolved nearly 50 years after it was described by Kawasaki in 1967. KD may result from an exposure of a genetically predisposed individual to a possible infectious environmental trigger. Up to 33 % of patients with KD have at least one concurrent infection at the time of diagnosis, but no correlation between a specific agent and the severity of the disease course has been identified [20, 21].

Clinical Manifestations

The diagnosis of KD is based on clinical criteria (Table 2) established by the Japanese Ministry of Health and adopted by the American Heart Association. If less than four of the principal features are present but two-dimensional echocardiography detects coronary artery abnormalities, patients are diagnosed with incomplete KD. Frequently, features of KD develop sequentially rather than simultaneously, which might result in misdiagnosis and treatment delay. In addition to the principal clinical findings, several other symptoms can be present, such as extreme irritability, arthritis, rhinorrhea, weakness, hydrops of the gallbladder, and mild anterior uveitis.

The clinical diagnosis can further be hindered in a subset of patients, mostly younger than 12 months of age or older than 5 years, with less than four of the principal features but with laboratory results or echocardiographic evidence that suggest the diagnosis of KD. These patients present with incomplete KD.

The variability in patient presentation should encourage clinicians to consider KD in any case of prolonged and unexplained fever.

Additional supplementary laboratory criteria can aid in establishing the correct diagnosis: decreased levels of albumin (<3 g/dl); increased C-reactive protein; increased erythrocyte sedimentation rate >40 mm/h; elevated alanine aminotransferase; leukocytosis >15,000/mm; normochromic, normocytic anemia for age; and sterile pyuria >10 white blood cells/mm^3.

Table 2 Diagnostic criteria for Kawasaki disease [22]

Fever (>39 °C) for at least 5 days	
AND at least four of the following five diagnostic features	
Polymorphous exanthema	
Bilateral bulbar conjunctival injection without exudate	
Changes in lips and oral cavity	Erythema, fissured cracked lips, strawberry tongue, or diffuse injection of oral and pharyngeal mucosae
Cervical lymphadenopathy	(>1.5 cm diameter), usually unilateral
Changes in extremities	Acute: erythema of palms and soles; edema of hands and feet
	Subacute: periungual peeling of fingers and toes (in the second and third week)
WITH exclusion of other diseases with similar clinical features	

The differential diagnosis of KD includes (1) various infections such as Epstein–Barr virus, adenovirus, echovirus, measles, toxic shock syndrome, scarlet fever, Rocky Mountain spotted fever, leptospirosis; (2) autoimmune diseases such as systemic-onset juvenile idiopathic arthritis or polyarteritis nodosa; and (3) juvenile mercury poisoning and adverse drug reactions including Stevens–Johnson disease.

The clinical course of the disease consists of four phases. In the acute phase, which lasts 1–2 weeks if untreated, children have a high spiking fever and principal symptomatic features. At this time, they may present with cardiac manifestation including valvulitis, pericarditis, and myocarditis. In the following subacute phase, children are at greatest risk of sudden death due to myocardial infarction. The subacute phase lasts approximately 2 weeks and is characterized by resolution of the fever. The third phase is the convalescent phase after cessation of symptoms and continues until acute-phase inflammatory markers return to normal serum levels. In the fourth, chronic phase, patients with coronary artery involvement require follow-up management (Figs. 3 and 4).

To reduce the risk of coronary artery involvement in later phases of the disease, diagnosis should be made in the acute stage so as to administer timely treatment and reduce inflammation [2, 4, 20, 21].

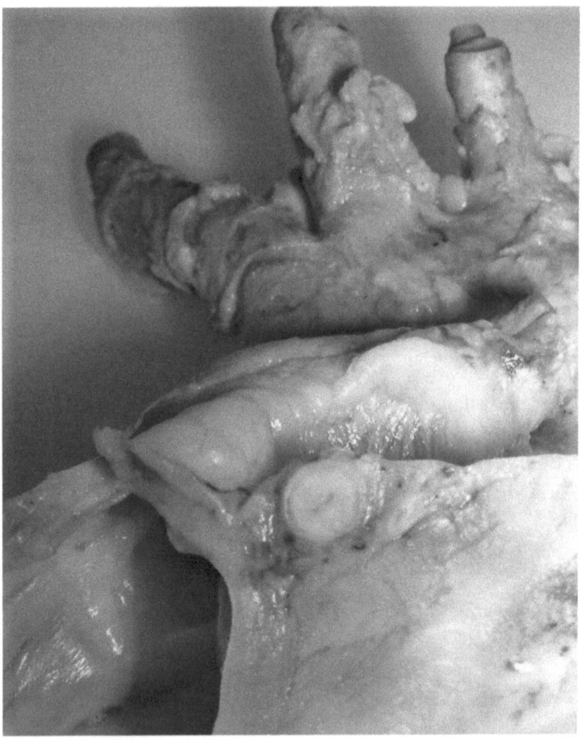

Fig. 3 Coronary artery vasculitis in a child with treatment-resistant Kawasaki disease and ischemic cardiomyopathy

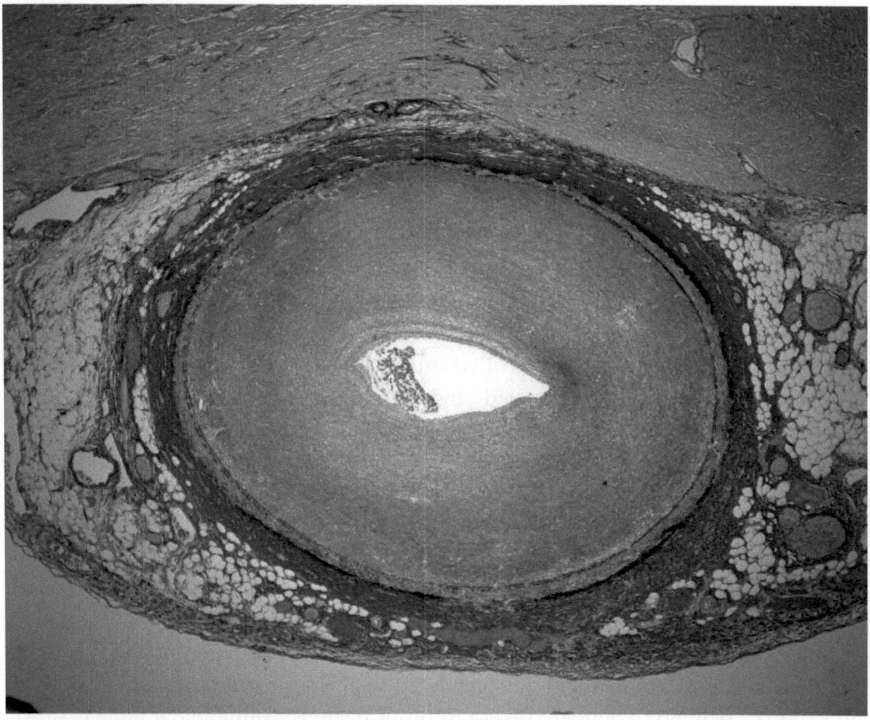

Fig. 4 Histological changes in coronary artery vasculitis in treatment-resistent Kawasaki disease

Treatment

The aim of acute-phase management in KD is to reduce inflammation, particularly inflammation in the coronary arteries and myocardium. Early treatment, before day 10 of the disease, with a single dose of intravenous immunoglobulin (IVIG) over 12 h at a dosage of 2 g/kg has been shown to greatly reduce the risk of coronary artery lesions. In addition to IVIG, high "anti-inflammatory" doses of acetylsalicylic acid (ASA) of 80–100 mg/kg/day in divided doses in the United States and of 30–50 mg/kg/day in divided doses in the United Kingdom and Japan are used in the acute phase. The dose of ASA is lowered to an "antiplatelet" dose (3–5 mg/kg/day) following defervescence. ASA is continued until inflammatory markers have returned to normal and there is no evidence of coronary artery lesions. However, a Cochrane Review concluded there is insufficient evidence in support of using ASA in the acute phase for coronary artery prevention [23].

Between 11 and 23 % of patients with KD treated with IVIG remain with a recurrent fever at least 36 h after the first IVIG infusion. IVIG-resistant patients are at higher risk of developing coronary artery aneurysms. There are several additional options to further decrease the ongoing inflammation, with a second dose of IVIG of 2 g/kg, intravenous GC pulse therapy, anti-tumor necrosis factor-α antibodies, and cytotoxic agents [24–27].

Early retrospective studies have shown that GCs were associated with an increased risk of coronary artery aneurysms. These results have almost certainly reflected selection bias as the sickest patients received steroids. Subsequent clinical trials that evaluated the use of GC in addition to IVIG have yielded seemingly confusing results [28, 29].

However, a recent meta-analysis provided convincing evidence that steroids combined with IVIG as initial treatment reduce the overall risk of coronary artery aneurysms in severe KD. The meta-analysis included nine clinical studies involving 1,011 patients (536 patients received IVIG and GC, 475 only IVIG). Six studies were prospective randomized controlled studies, one was a retrospective report, and two were nonrandomized controlled studies. They found that significantly fewer patients receiving IVIG and GC developed coronary artery aneurysms than those receiving IVIG alone. They also found no significant differences in frequency of severe adverse events between the steroid and nonsteroid treatment group. However, different studies used heterogeneous GC dosing regimens and it is difficult to translate the results into clinical practice [30].

Since 80 % of patients with KD respond to ASA and IVIG, and coronary artery aneurysms are most commonly seen in patients who fail to respond to IVIG, markers that would predict IVIG resistance are needed. If we could identify IVIG nonresponders, corticosteroids might be considered as an additional treatment to IVIG in this group of patients. There are several scoring systems available but none is sensitive or specific enough to be used in different populations. For example, the Kobayashi score, used by Japanese investigators in the RAISE study, had a low sensitivity for prediction of IVIG nonresponders in other studies [31, 32].

Eleftheriou et al. proposed that corticosteroids should be considered for: (1) IVIG-resistant patients with persistent inflammation and on-going fever of more than 48 h after receiving a first dose of IVIG of 2 mg/kg; (2) patients with features of more severe disease such as age younger than1 year, markers of severe inflammation, including persistently elevated CRP, liver dysfunction, hypoalbuminemia and anemia, features of hemophagocytic lymphohistiocytosis, and/or shock; and (3) patients with evolving coronary or peripheral aneurysms with on-going inflammation at presentation. It was suggested that intravenous preparations of prednisolone equivalent to 2 mg/kg should be used for 5–7 days, or until CRP normalizes. This should be followed by oral prednisolone weaning over 2–3 weeks. However, given the absence of strong evidence, some flexibility of steroid regimens for individual patients is suggested [31].

Polyarteritis Nodosa

The third most common childhood vasculitis in the Western hemisphere is polyarteritis nodosa (PAN). It is a necrotizing vasculitis of medium-sized muscular arteries and it accounts for approximately 3 % of childhood vasculitides. The EULAR/PReS classification criteria for PAN require evidence of inflammation of medium or small arteries either by histopathology or angiography and one of the following five criteria: involvement of skin, myalgia, hypertension, peripheral neuropathy, or renal involvement [22]. The etiology remains unclear; its association with hepatitis B, which is frequent in adult patients, is extremely rare in children.

The onset of the disease usually begins before 10 years of age. It starts with non-specific systemic symptoms with malaise, fever, weight loss, skin rash, myalgia, abdominal pain, and arthropathy. Laboratory markers of inflammation are usually elevated. PAN can affect a vessel and its supply anywhere in the body, although the lungs are typically spared. Owing to involvement of the medium-sized vessels, there can be ischemic symptoms of the affected organs such as ischemic heart pain, ischemic testicular involvement, focal neurological signs with hemiplegia, visual loss, and mononeuritis multiplex. Renal involvement can present as hematuria, proteinuria, and hypertension. Inflammation of the small arteries of the skin can present with variable skin lesions from livedo reticularis, purpura, or necrosis and possibly digital gangrene (Figs. 5 and 6). Characteristic features are painful subcutaneous nodules along the affected vessels [2, 33, 34].

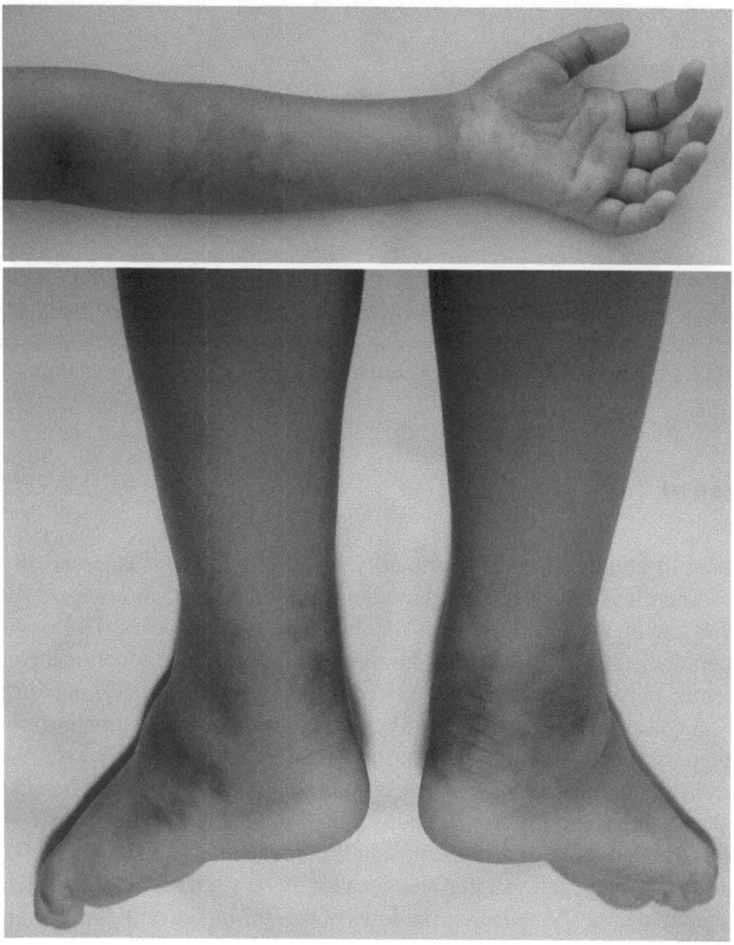

Fig. 5 Skin rash in a patient with polyarteritis nodosa

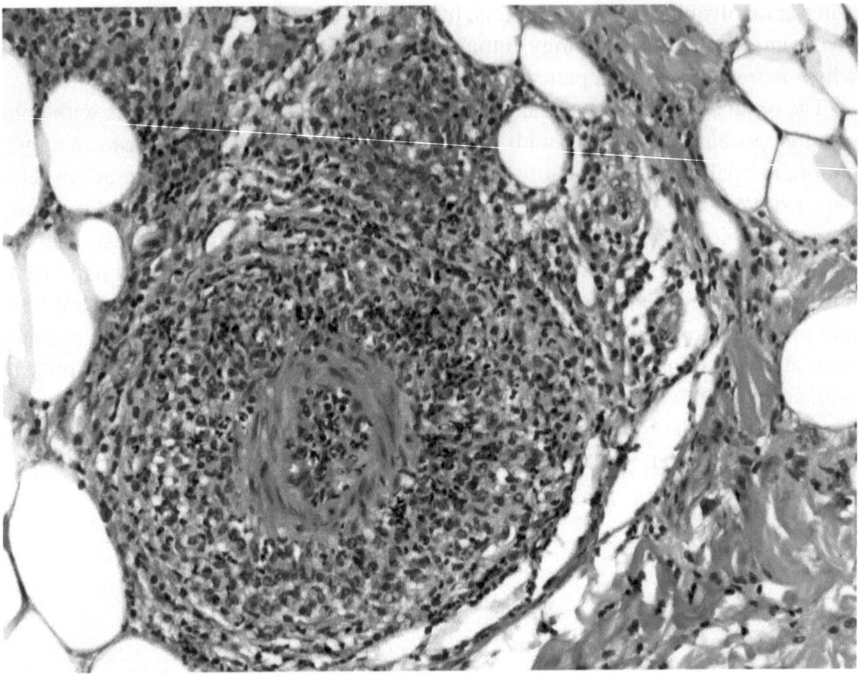

Fig. 6 Necrotizing arteritis in a child with polyarteritis nodosa

Cutaneous PAN is limited to the skin and musculoskeletal system and is often associated with antecedent streptococcal infection. It characteristically presents with fever, painful subcutaneous nodules, purpura, livedo reticularis, myalgias, arthralgias, and arthritis. Skin lesions are mostly present on the lower limbs.

Treatment

Treatment of childhood PAN is primarily based on clinical experience and adult studies. There have not been any randomized clinical trials to compare different induction and maintenance therapies for childhood systemic PAN. The cornerstone of induction therapy is GC with an additional cytotoxic agent. Induction therapy can be given as pulse intravenous methylprednisolone (30 mg/kg/day; maximal dose 1 g) for 3 consecutive days, followed by oral prednisolone with tapering, or orally with prednisolone (1–2 mg/kg/day) for 4 weeks with weaning over the next 6–8 weeks. Additional therapy with cyclophosphamide either oral (2 mg/kg/day) for 2–3 months or monthly intravenous pulses (500–1,000 mg/m^2) for 6 months may be warranted for induction therapy. In life-threatening situations, IVIG or plasmapheresis can be beneficial. For maintenance therapy after remission is achieved, daily or alternate-day prednisolone in doses of 0.3–0.7 mg/kg with oral azathioprine

(2 mg/kg/day) is used for up to 18 months. Alternatives to azathioprine include methotrexate or mycophenolate mofetil. Successful treatments with infliximab or rituximab have also been reported.

For treatment of cutaneous PAN the mainstay of therapy are NSAIDs or GCs in moderate doses. In cases of persistent or relapsing disease, steroid-sparing agents such as methotrexate, colchicine, and IVIG have been used. Owing to its connection with streptococcal infection, continuous penicillin prophylaxis might be beneficial [2, 4, 33, 34].

Takayasu Arteritis

TA is a granulomatous vasculitis of the aorta with its major branches, most commonly the subclavian, carotid, and renal arteries. Childhood TA is a disease of adolescence with a mean age of diagnosis at 13 years and is more common in female patients and in Asian populations. Consensus criteria of EULAR/PReS require as mandatory for classification of childhood TA typical angiographic abnormalities of the aorta or its main branches and pulmonary arteries plus one of five additional criteria: (1) pulse deficit or claudication, (2) blood pressure discrepancy in any limb, (3) an audible bruit, (4) hypertension, or (5) elevated acute-phase reactants [22].

Disease presents with nonspecific systemic features such as headaches, fevers, fatigue, back pain, myalgia and arthralgia, abdominal pain, and claudication of the extremities. Nearly 90 % of patients have hypertension at diagnosis. During the disease course, additional specific symptoms, determined by the distribution of vessel involvement, usually develop. With involvement of the aortic arch or its major branches signs of so-called supradiaphragmatic–aortic arch disease evolve: CNS symptoms with headache, ischemic strokes, cerebral aneurysms and seizures, claudication in the upper extremities, absent peripheral pulses, and cardiac manifestations such as cardiomyopathy, congestive heart disease, and valvular disease.

Infradiaphragmatic–midaortic syndrome often presents with hypertension, lower extremity claudication, abdominal bruits, and abdominal pain, which can be severe and intermittent with bloody diarrhea. With renal artery involvement, hypertension leads to encephalopathy [2, 4, 35, 36].

Treatment

Treatment of TA includes immunosuppression with corticosteroids, methotrexate, cyclophosphamide, or biological anti-inflammatory therapy for active vessel wall inflammation. Symptomatic treatment includes anticoagulation and antihypertensive therapy. Complications including various types of aortoarterial stenosis/occlusion or dilatation sometimes require surgical or endovascular management, such as percutaneous transluminal angioplasty [2, 4, 35]. In a recent single-center study of

21 patients with TA, 85.7 % of patients required prednisone therapy and 65.7 % of patients were treated with methotrexate. Ten of 21 patients required additional therapy to control the disease: infliximab, additional intravenous steroids, cyclophosphamide, anakinra, and etanercept. Eight (38.1 %) patients required surgical intervention [36].

ANCA-Associated Vasculitides

A group of vasculitides with predominantly pathological involvement of small and medium-sized blood vessels and association with antineutrophil cytoplasmic antibodies (ANCAs) are called the ANCA-associated vasculitides (AAV). They have overlapping clinical features with involvement of the lungs and kidneys. AAV are associated with a high frequency of disease- and treatment-related morbidities. Untreated AAV have near 100 % mortality with a mean survival of 5 months [2, 4]. In up to 60 % of patients, relapses occur. The three classic vasculitides are granulomatosis with polyangiitis (GPA, formerly known as Wegener's granulomatosis), microscopic polyangiitis, and eosinophilic granulomatosis with polyangiitis (EGPA, formerly Churg–Strauss syndrome) [2, 4].

Childhood-onset granulomatosis with polyangiitis primarily affects the upper and lower respiratory tract and kidneys. According to the EULAR/PReS guidelines, three out of six criteria are needed for classification of childhood-onset granulomatosis with polyangiitis: histopathological evidence of granulomatous inflammation; upper airway involvement, laryngo-tracheo-bronchial involvement; radiologic evidence of pulmonary involvement; ANCA positivity or renal involvement with proteinuria; hematuria, red blood cell cast; necrotizing pauci-immune glomerulonephritis. At diagnosis more than 90 % of patients have constitutional symptoms with fever, malaise, and weight loss, and 80 % have pulmonary manifestations that may include pulmonary hemorrhage, nodules, infiltrates, pleurisy, oxygen dependency, or respiratory failure. Involvement of the upper respiratory system with recurrent epistaxis, sinusitis, mastoiditis, nasal or oral ulcerations, nasal septum perforation, and subglottic stenosis are present in 80 % of the patients at diagnosis. Three quarters of patients have renal involvement. About 90 % of patients are ANCA-positive, with a great majority positive for cytoplasmic-ANCA (c-ANCA) or PR3-positive ANCA [37–39]. In a recent Japanese report of 23 patients with GPA, the proportion of MPO-ANCA-positive patients was higher, nearly one third, than in Western populations.

A necrotizing vasculitis that affects capillaries, venules, or arterioles most commonly in kidneys or lungs is called microscopic polyangiitis. In nearly all the patients described, constitutional symptoms of fever, weight loss, malaise, and arthralgias were present. Besides renal disease, which may include hypertension, hematuria, proteinuria, or even renal failure in one third of the patients, ischemic cerebral insults or necrotizing vasculitic lesions of the skin are present in 30 % of the patients. Three quarters of patients have perinuclear ANCA [2, 3, 38, 40].

Eosinophilic granulomatosis with polyangiitis (EGPA) affects small and medium-sized vessels primarily in severely asthmatic or allergic patients. There are no specific criteria for EGPA in children. The American College of Rheumatology classification criteria requires four of the following for diagnosis: (1) history of asthma, (2) history of allergies, (3) peripheral eosinophilia of 10 %, (4) mono- or polyneuropathy, (5) migratory pulmonary infiltrates, (6) paranasal sinus pain or radiographic opacities, or (7) biopsy demonstrating extravascular eosinophils. The most common features in children at diagnosis are asthma, pulmonary infiltrates, sinusitis, involvement of the skin with vasculitis rash, cardiac disease, gastrointestinal symptoms, polyneuropathy, and in rare cases kidney disease. Only 25 % of children with EGPA are ANCA-positive [2, 4, 41].

Treatment

Principles of treatment are similar for all AAV with induction and maintenance therapy. Treatment options have been mainly adapted from adult studies or case series. Treatment with a combination of GC and oral cyclophosphamide (CYC) has long been the standard of care for induction therapy and achieves remission in more than 90 % of patients. Before acceptance of this treatment protocol, the majority of severe cases in children were fatal. For GPA, the induction phase lasts for 3–6 months and includes prednisolone administered orally (1–2 mg/kg/day; max. 60 mg/day) in divided doses for 2–4 weeks followed by tapering. In extremely ill patients, 1–3 days of intravenous pulse methylprednisolone of 30 mg/kg/day is used. In addition to GCs, cyclophosphamide administered orally (2 mg/kg/day) or intravenous pulses of 0.5–1.0 g/m^2 monthly are used. Owing to significant treatment-related toxicities such as immunosuppression with serious infections, hemorrhagic cystitis, infertility, or development of malignancies and the high risk of relapse, different alternatives to CYC are being sought. Alternative immunosuppressants for less severe or steroid-dependent disease include methotrexate, azathioprine, mycophenolate mofetil, anti-tumor necrosis factor-α, and rituximab. Plasmapheresis can also provide additional benefits for most patients with severe disease.

For maintenance therapy, methotrexate, mycophenolate mofetil, or azathioprine for 18–24 months is used. Options for refractory disease include biological therapy: infliximab or rituximab and IVIg [2, 4, 40, 41].

Central Nervous System Vasculitis

Inflammatory disease of blood vessels in the brain in children not associated with vasculitis in other organs is called CNS vasculitis of childhood. It may be primary or secondary, associated with infection, rheumatic or systemic inflammatory disease, malignancies, metabolic disease, or medications and radiation therapy.

If the disease is diagnosed early, the inflammation and neurologic damage may be reversible. Based on the angiography findings, primary vasculitis is classified as: (1) large to medium-sized vessels primary central nervous system vasculitis (cPACNS) with abnormal angiography and (2) small vessel–cPACNS with normal angiography [42–45].

Patients with angiography-positive cPACNS typically present with focal neurologic symptoms and can have normal systemic inflammatory markers and cerebrospinal fluid analysis. Conventional angiography or magnetic resonance angiography demonstrates large or medium-sized vessel stenosis, occlusion, or bending. Focal areas of acute ischemia in a vascular distribution are found on magnetic resonance imaging. If new lesions appear within 3 months after diagnosis, cPACNS is further classified as progressive in contrast to nonprogressive disease. Patients with progressive disease more frequently have headaches, cognitive dysfunction, and behavioral changes.

Patients with diffuse or focal neurologic symptoms and angiography-negative cPACNS may have fever, malaise, and other systemic features at presentation. Usually the cerebrospinal fluid is pathological with increased opening pressure, pleocytosis, and elevated proteins; systemic inflammatory markers may be normal. Gray matter and white matter are involved unilaterally or bilaterally and changes are usually multifocal. To confirm the diagnosis, brain biopsy is needed and reveals lymphocytic nongranulomatous vasculitis [42–45].

Treatment

For nonprogressive cPACNS, treatment is controversial. It may include anticoagulation and corticosteroids, which can help to prevent recurrence and improve neurologic recovery.

Progressive cPACNS and angiography-negative cPACNS are treated aggressively with induction therapy for 6 months that includes cyclophosphamide (500–750 mg/m^2/month) and corticosteroids (2 mg/kg/day initially with tapering) followed by maintenance therapy with mycophenolate mofetil or azathioprine for 18 months [42–45].

References

1. Ozen S et al (2006) EULAR/PReS endorsed consensus criteria for the classification of childhood vasculitides. Ann Rheum Dis 65(7):936–941
2. Weiss PF (2012) Pediatric vasculitis. Pediatr Clin North Am 59(2):407–423
3. Batu ED, Ozen S (2012) Pediatric vasculitis. Curr Rheumatol Rep 14(2):121–129
4. Cassidy JT et al (2011) Textbook of pediatric rheumatology, 6th edn. Saunders Elsevier, Philadelphia

5. Gardner-Medwin JM et al (2002) Incidence of Henoch-Schonlein purpura, Kawasaki disease, and rare vasculitides in children of different ethnic origins. Lancet 360:1197–1202
6. Saulsbury FT (1999) Henoch-Schönlein purpura in children: report of 100 patients and review of the literature. Medicine (Baltimore) 78(6):395–409
7. Trnka P (2013) Henoch–Schönlein purpura in children. J Paediatr Child Health 49:995–1003
8. Trapani S et al (2005) Henoch Schonlein purpura in childhood: epidemiological and clinical analysis of 150 cases over a 5-year period and review of literature. Semin Arthritis Rheum 35(3):143–153
9. Kawasaki Y (2011) The pathogenesis and treatment of pediatric Henoch–Schönlein purpura nephritis. Clin Exp Nephrol 15:648–657
10. Huber AM et al (2004) A randomized, placebo-controlled trial of prednisone in early Henoch Schönlein purpura. BMC Med 2:7
11. Weiss PF et al (2007) Effects of corticosteroid on Henoch-Schönlein purpura: a systematic review. Pediatrics 120:1079–1087
12. Weiss PF et al (2009) Variation in inpatient therapy and diagnostic evaluation of children with Henoch Schönlein purpura. J Pediatr 155(6):812.e1–818.e1
13. Weiss PF et al (2010) Corticosteroids may improve clinical outcomes during hospitalization for Henoch-Schönlein purpura. Pediatrics 126(4):674–681
14. Szer IS (1999) Gastrointestinal and renal involvement in vasculitis: management strategies in Henoch-Schönlein purpura. Cleve Clin J Med 66:312–317
15. Ronkainen J et al (2006) Early prednisone therapy in Henoch-Schonlein purpura: a randomized, double-blind, placebo-controlled trial. J Pediatr 149:241–247
16. Chartapisak W et al (2009) Interventions for preventing and treating kidney disease in Henoch-Schönlein Purpura (HSP). Cochrane Database Syst Rev (3):CD005128
17. Jauhola O et al (2012) Outcome of Henoch-Schönlein purpura 8 years after treatment with a placebo or prednisone at disease onset. Pediatr Nephrol 27(6):933–939
18. Davin JC (2011) Henoch-Schonlein purpura nephritis: pathophysiology, treatment and future strategy. Clin J Am Soc Nephrol 6:679–689
19. Eleftheriou D et al (2009) Biologic therapy in primary systemic vasculitis of the young. Rheumatology 48:978–986
20. Jamieson N, Singh-Grewal D (2013) Kawasaki disease: a clinician's update. Int J Pediatr 2013:645391
21. Yim D et al (2013) An update on Kawasaki disease II: clinical features, diagnosis, treatment and outcomes. J Paediatr Child Health 49(8):614–623
22. Ozen S et al (2010) EULAR/PRINTO/PRES criteria for Henoch-Schönlein purpura, childhood polyarteritis nodosa, childhood Wegener granulomatosis and childhood Takayasu arteritis: Ankara 2008. Part II: final classification criteria. Ann Rheum Dis 69(5):798–806
23. Baumer JH et al (2006) Salicylate for the treatment of Kawasaki disease in children. Cochrane Database Syst Rev (4):CD004175
24. Brogan RJ et al (2009) Infliximab for the treatment of intravenous mmunoglobulin resistant Kawasaki disease complicated by coronary artery aneurysms: a case report. Pediatr Rheumatol Online J 7:3
25. Burns JC et al (2005) Infliximab treatment for refractory Kawasaki syndrome. J Pediatr 146:662–667
26. Oishi T et al (2008) Infliximab treatment for refractory Kawasaki disease with coronary artery aneurysm. Circ J 72:850
27. Weiss JE et al (2004) Infliximab as a novel therapy forrefractory Kawasaki disease. J Rheumatol 31:808–810
28. Inoue Y, Okada Y, Shinohara M et al (2006) A multicenter prospective randomized trial of corticosteroids in primary therapy for Kawasaki disease: clinical course and coronary martery outcome. J Pediatr 149:336–341
29. Newburger JW et al (2007) Randomized trial of pulsed corticosteroid therapy for primary treatment of Kawasaki disease. N Engl J Med 356:663–675

30. Chen S et al (2013) Intravenous immunoglobulin plus corticosteroid to prevent coronary artery abnormalities in Kawasaki disease: a meta-analysis. Heart 99(2):76–82
31. Eleftheriou D et al (2014) Management of Kawasaki disease. Arch Dis Child 99(1):74–83
32. Kobayashi T et al (2013) Efficacy of immunoglobulin plus prednisolone for prevention of coronary artery abnormalities in severe Kawasaki disease (RAISE study): a randomised, open-label, blinded-endpoints trial. Lancet 379(9826):1613–1620
33. Kawakami T (2012) A review of pediatric vasculitis with a focus on juvenile polyarteritis nodosa. Am J Clin Dermatol 13(6):389–398
34. Ozen S et al (2004) Juvenile polyarteritis: results of a multicenter survey of 110 children. J Pediatr 145:517–522
35. Cakar N et al (2008) Takayasu arteritis in children. J Rheumatol 35:913–919
36. Szugye HS et al (2014) Takayasu Arteritis in the pediatric population: a contemporary United States-Based Single Center Cohort. Pediatr Rheumatol 12:21
37. Akikusa JD et al (2007) Clinical features and outcome of pediatric Wegener's granulomatosis. Arthritis Rheum 57:837–844
38. Bohm M et al (2014) Clinical features of childhood granulomatosis with polyangiitis (wegener's granulomatosis). Pediatr Rheumatol Online J 12:18. doi:10.1186/1546-0096-12-18
39. Cabral DA et al (2009) Classification, presentation, and initial treatment of Wegener's granulomatosis in childhood. Arthritis Rheum 60:3413–3424
40. Sun L et al (2014) Clinical and pathological features of microscopic polyangiitis in 20 children. J Rheumatol 41(8):1712–1719
41. Zwerina J et al (2009) Churg-Strauss syndrome in childhood: a systematic literature review and clinical comparison with adult patients. Semin Arthritis Rheum 39:108–115
42. Benseler SM et al (2006) Primary central nervous system vasculitis in children. Arthritis Rheum 54:1291–1297
43. Calabrese LH et al (1992) Primary angiitis of the central nervous system: diagnostic criteria and clinical approach. Cleve Clin J Med 59:293–306
44. Gowdie P et al (2012) Primary and secondary central nervous system vasculitis. J Child Neurol 27(11):1448–1459
45. Iannetti L et al (2012) Recent understanding on diagnosis and management of central nervous system vasculitis. Child Clin Dev Immunol Vol. doi:10.1155/2012/698327

Corticosteroids in Pediatric-Onset SLE and Other Connective Tissue Diseases

Alexandre Belot

Introduction

Glucocorticoids (GCs) are potent anti-inflammatory drugs and have been widely used in many inflammatory diseases including connective tissue diseases (CTDs) in children. Although steroids are effective in controlling severe diseases such as juvenile systemic lupus erythematosus (SLE), it has become clear that they are associated with numerous side effects; it is now known that steroids should be used in GC-sparing regimens. In this chapter, we underscore the major impact of these drugs in disease control during the treatment of CTDs and we present new long-term therapeutic strategies aimed at reducing GC exposure. Steroids account for an important burden of the disease, especially in SLE where the cumulative steroid dose is considered damaging. SLE is the paradigm of autoimmune diseases; therefore, we review the impact of steroids in such conditions with a focus on juvenile SLE.

Pediatric SLE: Efficacy and Place of Steroids

Pediatric SLE Specificities

Pediatric-onset systemic lupus erythematosus (pSLE) is a rare multisystemic autoimmune disease that differs from adult-onset SLE by a more severe phenotype, especially renal and neurological involvement, and a greater contribution of genetic factors [1]. pSLE accounts for 10–15 % of all SLE cases. Renal involvement in

A. Belot, MD, PhD
Pediatric Rheumatology and Nephrology Department, Hôpital Femme Mère Enfant, Hospices Civils de Lyon, Université de Lyon, INSERM U1111, Lyon, France
e-mail: alexandre.belot@chu-lyon.fr

R. Cimaz (ed.), *Systemic Corticosteroids for Inflammatory Disorders in Pediatrics*, DOI 10.1007/978-3-319-16056-6_8

pSLE is more frequent than in its adult counterpart, with about 75 % of affected children experiencing a renal flare [2]. Lupus-associated damage occurring in a developing child can be devastating and can affect both physical and psychosocial factors.

However, in part as a consequence of increased life expectancy, patients with pSLE are now faced with considerable morbidity as a result of the sequelae of disease activity (notably renal and neuropsychiatric), medication side effects, and comorbid conditions such as recurrent infections, accelerated atherosclerosis, and hypertension. Such morbidity has a considerable impact on long-term quality of life, including problems related to the physical and psychological consequences of a chronic severe illness. In contrast to the damage in patients with adult-onset SLE, which is often steroid-related (e.g., atherosclerosis, cataracts, osteoporosis), damage in pSLE has been predominantly disease-related, highlighting the severity of the disease and the relative good tolerance of the children under aggressive treatment [2].

Corticosteroids are widely used for patients with lupus. In a study of steroid use in 549 patients of the Hopkins Lupus Cohort, only 11 % had never been treated with steroids [3]. Thus, the management of patients with pSLE is now aimed at lessening the development of permanent damage through screening for disease-associated complications and improved therapy.

Renal jSLE

The kidney is the main concern of pediatricians treating patients with SLE, since most children with SLE experience a renal flare over time. Failure to achieve and maintain remission of juvenile lupus nephritis (LN) reduces the overall 10-year survival by an estimated 15 % [4].

Treatment guidelines for proliferative juvenile LN suffer from a lack of dedicated trials [5]. The treatment of jSLE relies on off-label use of drugs approved for transplantation-related immunosuppression. Thus strategies are largely inspired from adult clinical trials and robust data on optimal dosing, efficacy, and safety are lacking. LN management is divided into induction treatment during the first 6 months and maintenance treatment thereafter.

For induction, oral mycophenolate mofetil (MMF) or intravenous (IV) cyclophosphamide (CTX) pulses are proposed to induce remission concomitantly with the chosen GC-dosing regimen. MMF is used at a dose of 600 mg/m^2 twice daily and has shown comparable efficacy to IV CTX for induction treatment of severe lupus nephritis in adults (ASPREVA Lupus Management Study) [6]. IV CTX can be used at various dosing regimens. The Euro-Lupus Nephritis Trial, performed with adult patients, demonstrated no difference between low-dose CTX (six infusions of 500 mg every 2 weeks) compared with the NIH-like regimen (six monthly pulses of 500–1,500 mg CTX followed by quarterly pulses titrated according to white blood cell count nadir to a maximum of 1,500 mg) in terms of treatment failure, achievement of renal remission, and occurrence of renal flares or adverse events [7].

GC dosing is based on physician experience and is not standardized. Interestingly, high-dose IV methylprednisolone pulses, but not oral steroids, have the potential to eliminate the interferon-α transcriptional signature in juvenile SLE by reducing circulating plasmacytoid dendritic cells [8]. These data suggest a benefit for high-dose IV GC. For induction treatment, the Childhood Arthritis and Rheumatology Research Alliance (CARRA) recommends three distinct regimens for steroid dosing (Fig. 1). All three strategies allow for the use of up to three high-dose methylprednisolone pulses (30 mg/kg/dose up to 1 g/dose). The objective of these strategies is to achieve a daily dose of oral glucocorticoids between 10 and 20 mg at the end of the first 6 months. A recent survey performed in CARRA sites found that only 43 % of children with LN were treated according to the recommendations of the CARRA group, underlining that LN management remains dramatically variable and additional effort is needed to standardize strategies, relying on controlled trials.

In maintenance therapies, steroids are usually continued at a low dose (2.5–5 mg/day). In the Hopkins Lupus Cohort, 57 % of patients with disease duration over 10 years have never discontinued steroids [3].

Other jSLE Lesions

Except for skin involvement, steroids remain the mainstay of treatment for other organ lesions in SLE. In the case of joint involvement, methotrexate can be proposed as a steroid-sparing agent. Azathioprine has been widely used to manage cytopenia, myositis, hepatitis, vasculitis, and nephritis [9]. MMF seems to be safe and has a similar efficacy to that in renal involvement [10]. Plasma exchange is of minor interest in SLE and may be occasionally useful in refractory antiphospholipid antibody syndrome.

SELECTION OF STEROID REGIMEN (Pick 1 of these 3)

Primarily ORAL*

Week (wk)	Daily dose >30kg (mg)	Daily dose ≤30mg
1-4	60-80	2mg/kg/d
5-6	60	2mg/kg/d
7-10	50	↓ by 5-10mg
11-12	40	↓ by 5mg
13-14	40	↓ by 5mg
15-18	30	↓ by 5mg
19-22	25	↓ by 2,5-5mg
23-24	20	↓ by 2,5-5mg

*Optional 3 day pulse in week 1 is permitted

OR

Primarily IV

Week	Steroid Pulses°	Daily dose >30kg (mg)	Daily dose ≤30mg
1	3/wk	20	10
2	1-3/wk	20	10
3	1-3/wk	20	10
4	1-3/wk	20	10
5-7	1-3/wk	20	10
8-11	1/mo	20	10
12-18	1/mo	15	7,5
19-24	1/mo	10	5

OR

MIXED oral / IV

Week	Steroid Pulses°	Daily dose >30kg (mg)	Daily dose ≤30mg
1	3/wk	60	1,5 mg/kg/d
2	1/month (mo)	60	1,5 mg/kg/d
3		50	1,2 mg/kg/d
4		40	1
5-8	1/mo	35	0,9
9-12	1/mo	30	0,8
13-16	1/mo	25	0,7
17-20	1/mo	20	0,6
21-24	1/mo	15	0,5

°Pulse methylprednisolone: 30mg/kg/dose ; maximum 1000mg

Fig. 1 Steroid regimen as proposed by the Childhood Arthritis and Rheumatology Research Alliance for juvenile systemic lupus erythematosus

Burden of Steroid Use in Pediatric-Onset SLE

General

Steroids constitute a significant source of morbidity in patients with lupus. Brunner et al. reported that children accumulated disease damage at almost twice the rate of adults and that long-term use of high-dose corticosteroids contributes to this disease damage [11].

In the Hopkins Lupus Cohort Study, corticosteroid-related damage was assessed in 539 patients including 18 with pediatric-onset SLE [3]. Osteoporotic fracture, coronary artery disease, cataracts, stroke, diabetes mellitus, and avascular necrosis were significantly associated with the cumulative corticosteroid dose. High-dose corticosteroid therapy contributes greatly to therapy-related damage in children.

Growth and Puberty

In a study by the Paediatric Rheumatology International Trials Organization (PRINTO), growth and puberty were evaluated in 1,015 children with SLE. Growth failure and delayed puberty were observed in 15.3 % and 11.3 %, respectively [12]. In another work, Rygg and colleagues highlighted that the negative effects of steroids on height and pubertal development were most pronounced in prepubertal and peripubertal children treated with over 400 mg/kg cumulative dose of GC [13].

Osteoporosis

Occurrence of osteopenia in patients with childhood-onset SLE has been well documented in studies assessing bone mineral density by dual-energy X-ray measurement [14–16]. Osteoporosis in jSLE is secondary to the cumulative effects of chronic inflammation, pubertal delay, renal failure, sustained steroid intake, and decreased sun exposure. The cumulative GC dosage is reported to be independently associated with decreased bone mass in patients with pSLE [16].

There are two leading mechanisms by which steroids induce osteopenia:

1. Osteoclastogenesis induction with increased expression of RANK ligand and lower expression of its decoy receptor osteoprotegerin
2. Inhibition of osteoblastogenesis by induction of osteoblast apoptosis and growth factor inhibition [17]

Keeping GC down to the lowest dose and using steroid-sparing agents are mandatory to avoid osteoporosis. In addition, vitamin D and calcium supplementation is required but guidelines are missing. Bisphosphonate use may be effective for restoring bone density, even in patients without fractures [18].

Dyslipidemia, Metabolic Syndrome, and Cardiovascular Complications

Steroids are considered a risk factor for atherosclerosis because they may induce hyperlipidemia, hyperglycemia, hypertension, and obesity in addition to being an independent risk factor for cardiovascular disease, which suggests that they may promote atherogenesis [19]. Given their lifelong exposure to atherogenic risk factors, children and adolescents with SLE are at a particularly high risk of developing premature atherosclerosis. The Atherosclerosis Prevention in Paediatric Lupus Erythematosus trial showed that atorvastatin may be effective in reducing carotid intima medial thickness progression in patients with pSLE in pubertal age with high C-reactive protein levels [20].

Infections

Mortality in the initial few years of disease is mainly associated with infections, resulting both from the use of immunosuppressants and from the SLE-related susceptibility to infections [21]. In the early phase of treatment or in the case of persisting lymphopenia, antibiotic prophylaxis with cotrimoxazole is advised.

Others

Hirsutism, moon facies, buffalo hump, acne, striae, and weight gain are additional side effects of steroids. These side effects have an impact on the self-esteem of adolescents and consequently on medication adherence.

New Drug Strategies in jSLE

In CTDs and especially in SLE, new drug regimens are now considered and aim at targeting more specifically the defective immune pathway and at sparing steroid use [22, 23].

Tacrolimus is a T cell-specific calcineurin inhibitor that prevents transcription of the early activation genes of interleukin-2 and suppresses T cell-induced activation of cytokines. Recent studies in adult-onset SLE have found tacrolimus to be effective and relatively safe [24–26]. Multitarget therapies including steroids, low-dose tacrolimus, and mizoribine – an inhibitor of purine nucleotide synthesis similar to MMF – have been tested in children with lupus nephritis (Class III, IV, and/or V) with good efficacy [27].

In renal transplantation, the use of induction regimens with depleting antibodies has allowed steroid dosing to be avoided or dramatically reduced. The LUNAR study, a randomized controlled trial, has compared high-dose steroids plus MMF with high-dose steroids plus MMF plus rituximab. This study did not reveal any benefit of rituximab as an add-on therapy [28]. Lighstone and colleagues in an observational single-center study proposed the rituxilup protocol, using rituximab and methylprednisolone on day 1 and day 15, associated with daily MMF treatment with a good response [29, 30]. This study and others suggest that rituximab may be used as a steroid-sparing strategy in lupus nephritis. Further controlled studies including pediatric patients are ongoing.

Belimumab is an antibody directed against B cell-activating factor. Although it has been approved by the Food and Drug Administration for treatment of active non-renal adult-onset SLE, data in children are lacking [31, 32]. It may represent an interesting add-on therapy in juvenile SLE. Current clinical trials assessing safety and pharmacokinetics are ongoing in children.

Steroids in Other CTDs

Juvenile Dermatomyositis

Treatments for juvenile dermatomyositis or other inflammatory myopathies have not been assessed in randomized controlled trials [33]. As in pSLE, treatment relies on steroids. In daily practice, steroids are often used for the first 2 years of treatment. Early initiation of high-dose steroids seems to be associated with a decreased incidence of calcinosis [34]. In addition, gut vasculitis may impact on oral steroid absorption, and some physicians treat patients with repeated pulses of high-dose IV methylprednisolone in addition to low-dose daily oral corticosteroid as this strategy can be cost-effective and may be associated with an earlier remission [35]. Delayed or inadequate corticosteroid treatment is one of the most important predictors of poor outcome with decreased bone density and chronic active skin lesions [15, 34, 36]. Initial treatment plans have also been proposed by the CARRA for juvenile dermatomyositis (Fig. 2).

Mixed Connective Tissue Disease

Mixed connective tissue disease is rare in children, accounting for less than 1 % of pediatric rheumatology patients in one series [37]. Steroids were used in 71 % of patients, depending on the affected organs [38]. Currently, there are no guidelines on the steroid regimen and most of the strategies are linked to the clinical spectrum/overlapping symptoms.

SELECTION OF STEROID REGIMEN for Juvenile Dermatomyositis in the first month

Treatment A				Treatement B					Treatement C	
IV MP°	MTX*	Oral steroids		IV MP°	MTX*	Oral steroids	IV Ig		MTX*	Oral steroids
One pulse a day for 3 days, then one/week (optional)	Weekly	2mg/kg/d	OR	One pulse a day for 3 days, then one/week (optional)	Weekly	2mg/kg/d	2g/kg every 2 weeks	OR	Weekly	2mg/kg/d

°Pulse methylprednisolone: 30mg/kg/dose ; maximum 1000mg, *MTX: 15mg/m2 or 1mg/kg once weekly

Fig. 2 First 4 weeks of treatment in juvenile dermatomyositis

Juvenile Scleroderma

There are two main forms of the disease: juvenile localized scleroderma (JLS) and juvenile systemic sclerosis. The steroid administration mode highly depends on the specialty of the provider. In JLS, dermatologists prescribe topical steroids in 68 % and methotrexate in 4 % of patients, whereas rheumatologists conversely treat with local steroids in 4 % of cases and methotrexate in 38.8 % [39]. The CARRA group also proposed three distinct steroid regimens for JLS [40]: one regimen with methotrexate only, a second regimen with methotrexate + IV corticosteroids (either three consecutive daily doses/month for 3 months or one pulse/week × 12 weeks), and a third with methotrexate and oral prednisone (from 2 mg/kg/day initially to 12.5 % of initial dose at week 24).

Conclusions and Perspectives

Overall survival in CTDs has improved during the past few decades. Steroids are particularly effective in controlling inflammation during disease flares and for this reason they remain the cornerstone of treatment of CTDs. Alternative therapies, such as multitarget strategies or targeted therapies may help to decrease cumulative exposure to steroids, especially for remission induction. Treatments are mostly empirical and controlled trials in pediatric-onset CTDs are lacking. Further studies are highly warranted.

References

1. Belot A, Cimaz R (2012) Monogenic forms of systemic lupus erythematosus: new insights into SLE pathogenesis. Pediatr Rheumatol Online J 10:21
2. Watson L et al (2012) Disease activity, severity, and damage in the UK juvenile-onset systemic lupus erythematosus cohort. Arthritis Rheum 64:2356–2365

3. Zonana-Nacach A, Barr SG, Magder LS, Petri M (2000) Damage in systemic lupus erythematosus and its association with corticosteroids. Arthritis Rheum 43:1801–1808
4. Marks SD, Sebire NJ, Pilkington C, Tullus K (2007) Clinicopathological correlations of paediatric lupus nephritis. Pediatr Nephrol 22:77–83
5. Mina R et al (2012) Consensus treatment plans for induction therapy of newly diagnosed proliferative lupus nephritis in juvenile systemic lupus erythematosus. Arthritis Care Res 64:375–383
6. Appel GB et al (2009) Mycophenolate mofetil versus cyclophosphamide for induction treatment of lupus nephritis. J Am Soc Nephrol 20:1103–1112
7. Houssiau FA et al (2002) Immunosuppressive therapy in lupus nephritis: the Euro-Lupus Nephritis Trial, a randomized trial of low-dose versus high-dose intravenous cyclophosphamide. Arthritis Rheum 46:2121–2131
8. Guiducci C et al (2010) TLR recognition of self nucleic acids hampers glucocorticoid activity in lupus. Nature 465:937–941
9. Aggarwal A, Srivastava P (2015) Childhood onset systemic lupus erythematosus: how is it different from adult SLE? Int J Rheum Dis 18:182–191 n/a–n/a. doi:10.1111/1756-185X.12419
10. Dooley MA et al (2011) Mycophenolate versus azathioprine as maintenance therapy for lupus nephritis. N Engl J Med 365:1886–1895
11. Brunner HI, Silverman ED, To T, Bombardier C, Feldman BM (2002) Risk factors for damage in childhood-onset systemic lupus erythematosus: cumulative disease activity and medication use predict disease damage. Arthritis Rheum 46:436–444
12. Gutiérrez-Suárez R et al (2006) A proposal for a pediatric version of the Systemic Lupus International Collaborating Clinics/American College of Rheumatology Damage Index based on the analysis of 1,015 patients with juvenile-onset systemic lupus erythematosus. Arthritis Rheum 54:2989–2996
13. Rygg M et al (2012) A longitudinal PRINTO study on growth and puberty in juvenile systemic lupus erythematosus. Ann Rheum Dis 71:511–517
14. Stagi S et al (2014) Comparison of bone mass and quality determinants in adolescents and young adults with juvenile systemic lupus erythematosus (JSLE) and juvenile idiopathic arthritis (JIA). Lupus. doi:10.1177/0961203314543916
15. Alsufyani KA et al (2005) Bone mineral density in children and adolescents with systemic lupus erythematosus, juvenile dermatomyositis, and systemic vasculitis: relationship to disease duration, cumulative corticosteroid dose, calcium intake, and exercise. J Rheumatol 32:729–733
16. Lilleby V et al (2005) Frequency of osteopenia in children and young adults with childhood-onset systemic lupus erythematosus. Arthritis Rheum 52:2051–2059
17. Lilleby V (2007) Review: bone status in juvenile systemic lupus erythematosus. Lupus 16:580–586
18. Rudge S et al (2005) Effects of once-weekly oral alendronate on bone in children on glucocorticoid treatment. Rheumatology (Oxford) 44:813–818
19. Petri M, Lakatta C, Magder L, Goldman D (1994) Effect of prednisone and hydroxychloroquine on coronary artery disease risk factors in systemic lupus erythematosus: a longitudinal data analysis. Am J Med 96:254–259
20. Ardoin SP et al (2014) Secondary analysis of APPLE study suggests atorvastatin may reduce atherosclerosis progression in pubertal lupus patients with higher C reactive protein. Ann Rheum Dis 73:557–566
21. Vachvanichsanong P, Dissaneewate P, McNeil E (2011) Twenty-two years' experience with childhood-onset SLE in a developing country: are outcomes similar to developed countries? Arch Dis Child 96:44–49
22. Cimaz R (2012) Pediatric rheumatic disease: treating lupus nephritis in children–is there a gold standard? Nat Rev Rheumatol 8:192–193
23. Ranchin B, Fargue S (2007) New treatment strategies for proliferative lupus nephritis: keep children in mind! Lupus 16:684–691

24. Bao H et al (2008) Successful treatment of class V+IV lupus nephritis with multitarget therapy. J Am Soc Nephrol 19:2001–2010
25. Lanata CM, Mahmood T, Fine DM, Petri M (2010) Combination therapy of mycophenolate mofetil and tacrolimus in lupus nephritis. Lupus 19:935–940
26. Cortés-Hernández J, Torres-Salido MT, Medrano AS, Tarrés MV, Ordi-Ros J (2010) Long-term outcomes–mycophenolate mofetil treatment for lupus nephritis with addition of tacrolimus for resistant cases. Nephrol Dial Transplant 25:3939–3948
27. Tanaka H et al (2014) Efficacy of mizoribine-tacrolimus-based induction therapy for pediatric lupus nephritis. Lupus 23:813–818
28. Rovin BH et al (2012) Efficacy and safety of rituximab in patients with active proliferative lupus nephritis: the Lupus Nephritis Assessment with Rituximab study. Arthritis Rheum 64:1215–1226
29. Condon MB et al (2013) Prospective observational single-centre cohort study to evaluate the effectiveness of treating lupus nephritis with rituximab and mycophenolate mofetil but no oral steroids. Ann Rheum Dis 72:1280–1286
30. Weidenbusch M, Römmele C, Schröttle A, Anders H-J (2013) Beyond the LUNAR trial. Efficacy of rituximab in refractory lupus nephritis. Nephrol Dial Transplant 28:106–111
31. Furie R et al (2011) A phase III, randomized, placebo-controlled study of belimumab, a monoclonal antibody that inhibits B lymphocyte stimulator, in patients with systemic lupus erythematosus. Arthritis Rheum 63:3918–3930
32. Hui-Yuen JS et al (2014) A23: favorable response to belimumab in childhood-onset systemic lupus erythematosus. Arthritis Rheum 66 Suppl 11:S37, Hoboken
33. Feldman BM, Rider LG, Reed AM, Pachman LM (2008) Juvenile dermatomyositis and other idiopathic inflammatory myopathies of childhood. Lancet 371:2201–2212
34. Bowyer SL, Blane CE, Sullivan DB, Cassidy JT (1983) Childhood dermatomyositis: factors predicting functional outcome and development of dystrophic calcification. J Pediatr 103:882–888
35. Klein-Gitelman MS, Waters T, Pachman LM (2000) The economic impact of intermittent high-dose intravenous versus oral corticosteroid treatment of juvenile dermatomyositis. Arthritis Care Res 13:360–368
36. Rouster-Stevens KA et al (2007) RANKL: osteoprotegerin ratio and bone mineral density in children with untreated juvenile dermatomyositis. Arthritis Rheum 56:977–983
37. Michels H (1997) Course of mixed connective tissue disease in children. Ann Med 29:359–364
38. Mier RJ et al (2005) Pediatric-onset mixed connective tissue disease. Rheum Dis Clin North Am 31:483–496, vii
39. Johnson W, Jacobe H (2012) Morphea in adults and children cohort II: patients with morphea experience delay in diagnosis and large variation in treatment. J Am Acad Dermatol 67:881–889
40. Li SC et al (2012) Development of consensus treatment plans for juvenile localized scleroderma: a roadmap toward comparative effectiveness studies in juvenile localized scleroderma. Arthritis Care Res 64:1175–1185

24. Bao H et al. 2008 Successful treatment of class V+IV lupus nephritis with multitarget therapy. J Am Soc Nephrol 19:2001–2010
25. Dooley GM, Mahmood ... [illegible] (2010) Combination therapy of mycophenolate mofetil and tacrolimus in lupus nephritis. Lupus 19:935–940
26. Cortés-Hernández J, ... [illegible], Bucas MV, ... [illegible] (2010) Long-term outcomes – mycophenolate mofetil treatment for lupus nephritis with addition of tacrolimus for resistant cases. Nephrol Dial Transplant 25:3939–3948
27. [illegible] (2005) [illegible] multitarget therapy [illegible] lupus nephritis. Lupus 14:[illegible]–818
[illegible]

Glucocorticoids in Pediatric Gastrointestinal Disorders

Sara De Iudicibus, Stefano Martelossi, and Giuliana Decorti

Pediatric Inflammatory Bowel Disease

Inflammatory bowel diseases (IBDs) are the most frequent chronic gastrointestinal disorders in pediatric age. They include two disease entities – Crohn's disease (CD) and ulcerative colitis (UC) – which, although different in their pathogenesis, show common clinical characteristics such as chronic inflammation at different levels of the gastrointestinal tract and alternation between active and inactive phases. The incidence of IBD is increasing in recent years, particularly among children and adolescents, and it is currently estimated that 20–30 % of patients with IBD experience the onset of symptoms when they are under 20 years of age [1–3]. In childhood, IBDs are generally more extended, more severe, and progress more rapidly than in adulthood. Moreover, therapy in children with IBD is more aggressive than in adults: Indeed, about 80 % of children need steroids, and about 30 % are subjected to an intestinal resection during a 5-year follow-up. Quality of life is severely affected in IBD, especially for pediatric patients, owing to the chronic character of the disease that implies frequent hospitalizations and aggressive therapies, with a significant risk of side effects and a considerable impact on health care costs. IBD can result in loss of education and difficulty in gaining employment or insurance; overall, 15 % of patients with IBD are unable to work after 5–10 years of disease. Depressive disorders and low social functioning are also common among these patients, and the disease can also cause growth failure or retarded sexual development in young people [4–7]. It was recently reported that the mean individual annual costs in European countries amount to US$6,000 for CD and $4,600 for UC, and pediatric cases cost even more than adult ones [8].

S. De Iudicibus (✉) • S. Martelossi
Department of Pediatrics,
Institute for Maternal and Child Health IRCCS Burlo Garofolo, Trieste 34137, Italy
e-mail: sadeiu@libero.it

G. Decorti
Department of Life Sciences, University of Trieste, Trieste 34127, Italy

R. Cimaz (ed.), *Systemic Corticosteroids for Inflammatory Disorders in Pediatrics*, DOI 10.1007/978-3-319-16056-6_9

Induction of Remission with Glucocorticoids

UC and CD are complex disorders characterized by a wide variation in clinical characteristics. To date, treatment goals in IBD are evolving beyond the control of symptoms toward the tight control of objectively measured gastrointestinal inflammation [9]. Glucocorticoids (GCs) have been used to treat patients with active IBD for nearly 50 years [10], and despite the introduction of highly effective biological drugs in therapy, in patients with moderate to severe IBD GCs are still used to induce remission. In UC with pancolic localization, GCs are the gold standard for treatment and are always the first choice. In CD with pediatric onset, the first-line therapy is exclusive enteral nutrition: It is generally used for induction of remission and is achieved within 6–8 weeks of exclusive liquid feeding with either elemental or polymeric formulae [11]. In children with moderate to severe active luminal CD, oral corticosteroids are recommended for inducing remission if exclusive enteral nutrition is not an option.

In addition, in cases of CD with colic localization and with extraintestinal manifestations or severe prognosis (perianal disease, extensive disease), today the trend is to use immediately anti-tumor necrosis factor-α biologic agents, in an attempt to change the natural history of the disease.

When GCs are needed, oral prednisone is the agent of choice, and the standard treatment consists in administration of prednisone 1–2 mg/kg/day for 2–3 weeks (maximum dose 50 mg/day) and subsequent dose tapering every week. Different clinical responses have been observed with these agents in IBD; indeed, up to 90 % of pediatric patients have a rapid improvement of symptoms when a prednisone equivalent of 1–2 mg/kg/day is given [12]. After 1 year, only 55 % of early steroid-treated patients are still in remission and are deemed steroid-responsive, while around 38 % of patients are not able to discontinue the therapy and experience an increase in disease activity when the dose is reduced or during the first year after discontinuation; these patients are considered steroid-dependent. Seven percent of subjects are resistant and do not respond to GC therapy [13, 14]. In adults, steroid-dependence is more restrictive than in children, and is defined as the inability to taper GCs to less than 10 mg/day within 3 months of starting steroids without recurrent disease, or as the occurrence of relapse within 3 months of stopping GCs.

In children with mild to moderate ileocecal CD, budesonide may be used as an alternative to systemic corticosteroids for induction of remission [15]. The drug is taken orally and released in the distal small bowel and proximal colon; acting locally, this agent causes fewer systemic side effects. In subjects with mild to moderate ileal–right colonic disease, 9 mg of budesonide daily was superior to 4 g/day of mesalamine in inducing remission at 8 weeks (69 % vs. 45 %) and 16 weeks (62 % vs. 36 %) [16, 17].

Side Effects Associated with Glucocorticoid Treatment

The risks for adverse effects of GCs are related to the dose and the length of treatment, but sensitivity among individuals may vary greatly [15].

Growth failure and delayed puberty are present in a great proportion of children with IBD as a consequence of the disease and require particular attention; these conditions may be primarily related to malnutrition and to the strong inflammatory reaction occurring during active disease [18, 19, 20]. Furthermore, GC therapy, although efficient in inducing remission, clearly shows deleterious effects on growth. The mechanisms by which GCs suppress growth are complex. Pediatric patients with active IBD already have abnormal bone turnover [21], but GC exposure leads to promotion of osteoblast and osteocyte apoptosis, resulting in reduced bone formation, and these effects end with GC withdrawal [22, 23]. In addition, emerging evidence suggests these conditions could increase the risk of vertebral fractures in pediatric patients with IBD treated with GCs [24], but the minimum dose and duration of therapy that may cause damage to bones and fractures in children with IBD are currently unknown. Conversely, the negative effects of GCs on bone may be offset by their capacity to reduce inflammation.

Another important side effect observed in pediatric patients with IBD treated with GCs is adrenal suppression. This is a condition in which adrenal glands do not produce adequate amounts of cortisol when GC therapy is stopped, and is caused by suppression of the hypothalamic–pituitary–adrenal (HPA) axis by the circulating exogenous GCs [25, 26]. Sidoroff and colleagues [25] showed that at least one fifth of pediatric patients with IBD present with abnormal or even undetectable serum cortisol values at the end of systemic GC treatment. For patients with low levels of cortisol, hydrocortisone substitution was introduced until observing cortisol values within normal range.

Other common side effects include acne, facial hair growth, weight gain, and rounding of the face, and most of these will decrease when the drug is tapered down and discontinued. These side effects can trouble the patient, particularly female patients and/or adolescents, and can influence negatively compliance to therapy, especially in the case of repeated cycles of treatment.

Glucocorticoid Resistance in IBD

In inflammatory diseases, GC resistance or dependence is particularly frequent. As reported in the previous section, clinical studies in pediatric patients with IBD have shown that up to 90–95 % of subjects had a rapid improvement of symptoms when prednisone is given, but 5–10 % of patients still showed active disease [12, 27]. In addition, around 40 % of patients are considered dependent: They are not able to discontinue the therapy and experience an increase in disease activity when the dose is reduced or they relapse within 1 year of treatment suspension.

The phenomenon of GC resistance in chronic inflammatory diseases should be separated from the rare familial condition of primary generalized GC resistance, for which the name Chrousos syndrome was recently proposed [28]: This is a rare, sporadic, or familiar syndrome caused by mutations in the *NR3C1* (nuclear receptor subfamily 3, group C, member 1) gene. The disease is characterized by target tissue insensitivity to GCs due to reduction or lack of functional GC receptors and by compensatory elevation in adrenocorticotropic hormone (ACTH). This results in an increased secretion of cortisol, albeit in the absence of signs of Cushing's syndrome, as well as of other adrenal hormones with mineralocorticoid and androgenic activities, which is responsible for the main symptoms (hypertension and signs of hyperandrogenism). As mentioned, however, this syndrome is extremely rare, and no cases in patients with IBD have been described in the literature [29].

The most common forms of resistance observed in chronic inflammatory conditions, and in IBD in particular, may occur at several levels in the complex GC mechanism of action.

Molecular Mechanism of GC Action

The effects of GCs are mediated by the glucocorticoid receptor (GR)-α, a member of the nuclear receptor superfamily of ligand-dependent transcription factors [30, 31]. The human GR gene (*NR3C1*) is located on chromosome 5q31.3 and consists of nine coding exons [32]. Alternative splicing of exon 9 generates two receptor isoforms, GR-α and GR-β [33–36]. GR-β is not able to bind GCs, resides constitutively in the nucleus of cells, has a longer half-life than GR-α, and does not transactivate GC-inducible reporter genes [37]. It has been suggested [38, 39] that cell-specific expression and function of GR isoforms may explain the tissue- and individual-selective actions of GCs.

The function of GR is conditioned by chaperone and cochaperone proteins that form a molecular heterocomplex with the GR itself [40, 41], required for proper ligand binding, receptor activation, and transcription: Abnormalities in proteins that make up the heterocomplex may contribute to altered GC responsiveness [42, 43]. Several studies have demonstrated differences in the heterocomplex gene expression profiles in steroid-resistant versus steroid-responsive patients, but it is not clear if this different expression is the cause of the variability in response or the consequence of GC treatment [28, 44–48]. After GC binding and dissociation from heterocomplex proteins, the GR translocates into the nucleus; translocation is mediated by specific nuclear transport factors that belong to the importin-β family of nuclear transporters, and in particular by importin 13 [49]. The activated receptor then binds as homodimer to two palindromic DNA-binding sites, the so-called GC-responsive elements (GREs), localized in the promoter region of target genes [50–52]. As a consequence of DNA binding, GCs can induce transactivation and transrepression processes: Binding to positive GREs leads to activation of the transcription of anti-inflammatory [e.g., interleukin-10 (IL-10), annexin 1] as well as of regulator proteins involved in metabolic processes (e.g., enzymes of gluconeogenesis) [53–55].

The second mechanism of GC action is transrepression [56], which leads to a reduced expression of immune-regulatory and proinflammatory proteins such as cytokines (IL-1, IL-2, IL-6, tumor necrosis factor-α) and prostaglandins [57], and is

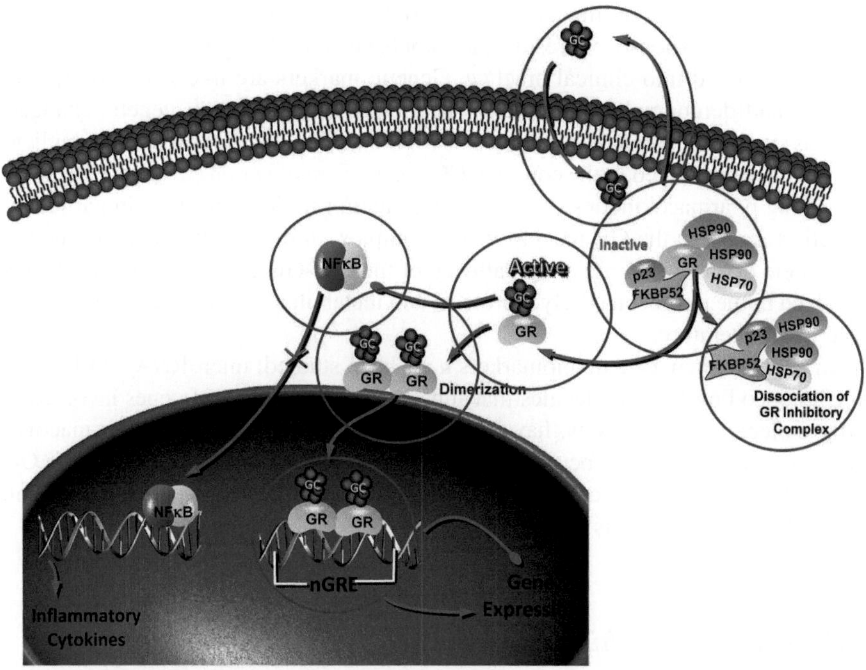

Fig. 1 Molecular mechanism of glucocorticoid action. *GR* glucocorticoid receptor, *GC* glucocorticoid, *HSP* heat-shock protein, *FKBP* FK506-binding protein, *NF-kB* nuclear factor-kB

believed to be responsible for the majority of beneficial anti-inflammatory effects. Furthermore, GRE-independent mechanisms of transrepression also exist: The GR physically interacts with activator protein-1 [58], nuclear factor-kB [59], and signal transducers and activators of transcription [60].

Steroid hormones can also regulate gene expression posttranscriptionally, by destabilizing mRNAs [61]. In addition, these hormones can induce rapid nongenomic effects within the cytoplasm; for example, they induce the release of Src kinase from the GR heterocomplex, resulting in lipocortin activation and inhibition of arachidonic acid release [62, 63], and they alter cytoplasmic ion content [64, 65] (Fig. 1).

Genetic and Epigenetic Predictors of GC Response

Given the high incidence of suboptimal response, associated with a significant number of side effects, the identification of subjects who are most likely to respond poorly to these agents seems extremely important. However, the mechanisms of steroid resistance and/or dependence are scarcely understood and there is presently no means to predict the response in advance.

Demographic and/or clinical markers [10, 66, 67] have been examined in correlation with GC response, but results have not been consistently replicated and could not be translated into clinical practice. Genetic markers are likely to complement clinical and demographic predictors. Phenotypes resulting from genetic changes, such as single nucleotide polymorphisms (SNPs), deletions, insertions, and duplications in genes involved in the complex GC mechanism of action can markedly influence drug pharmacokinetics or alter efficacy and/or toxicity profiles; in particular, genetic variants in the GR receptor heterocomplex, in the proinflammatory mediators in the downstream signaling pathway of the GC–GR complex, and in proteins involved in the extrusion (P-glycoprotein) and metabolism of GCs have been evaluated in the literature.

In addition, new genetic biomarkers have been studied: microRNAs (miRNAs), small noncoding RNA molecules that suppress the expression of genes involved in drug molecular mechanisms, have emerged as a promising field of pharmacogenomic research. Here we focus our attention on GR, which has a central role in GC molecular mechanisms, considering polymorphisms in its gene and the expression of miRNAs involved in its regulation.

GR Gene Polymorphisms

The human GR gene, *NR3C1* (nuclear receptor subfamily 3, group C, member 1; Nuclear Receptor Nomenclature Committee, 1999), is located on chromosome 5q31.3 and includes nine exons [32]. Polymorphisms of this gene may impair the formation of the GC–GR complex and subsequently alter transactivation and/or transrepression processes that have been related to increased [68] or decreased [69] sensitivity to endogenous cortisol.

The *TthIIII* (rs10052957), ER22/23EK (rs6189/rs6190), GR-9β (rs6198), N363S (rs6195), and *Bcl*I (rs41423247) polymorphisms have been the most studied and have been associated with differences in metabolic parameters and body composition as well as with autoimmune and cardiovascular disease. These genetic variants have also been related to changes in GC sensitivity [70] and may therefore account for the variability in the response to GC therapy. Although very few studies deal with the mechanisms, it is usually assumed that NR3C1 polymorphisms lead to a modified GR transcript.

TthIIII (rs10052957) is a restriction fragment length polymorphism (RFLP) caused by a C>T change in the GR gene promoter region; it is located in a large intron of approximately 27 kb, 3,807 bp upstream of the GR start site [71]. This polymorphism has been associated with elevated diurnal cortisol levels and with a reduced cortisol response to 1 mg dexamethasone (DEX), as well as lower insulin and cholesterol levels [68]. Other studies suggest that this polymorphism has a biological role mainly in association with other GR polymorphisms, forming haplotypes [72], but to date it has not been correlated with clinical response to GCs in patients with IBD, neither alone nor in haplotype.

The ER22/23EK polymorphisms (rs6189+rs6190) are located in the N-terminal transactivation domain of the GR and involve two nucleotide changes in codons 22 and 23 of exon 2 (GAG AGG to GAA AAG), which change the amino acid sequence from glutamic acid–arginine (E-R) to glutamic acid–lysine (E-K). Since the polymorphism is located in the transactivation domain, the amino acid change might affect the receptor's tertiary structure, influencing the transactivational and/or transrepressional activity on target genes [73]. An association with higher post-DEX cortisol levels and less cortisol suppression after a 1 mg DEX suppression test in ER22/23EK carriers has been shown. In addition, the polymorphism is associated with a better metabolic and cardiovascular health profile and an increased survival [68, 69]. In a study considering the role of ER22/23EK in the variability of clinical response to GCs in IBD, no association was found between the ER22/23EK polymorphism and GC response in 119 pediatric patients [74]. These polymorphisms have been also studied in adult patients with IBD, but no correlation has been observed with GC-resistant phenotype, even when dividing patients into UC and CD groups [75].

GR-9β (rs6198) is an A to G nucleotide substitution located in the 3'-UTR of exon 9β, the terminal exon of the mRNA of the β isoform (nucleotide 3669 in X03348; rs 6198). The A to G nucleotide substitution is located in an ATTTA motif (changing it to GTTTA). This ATTTA motif is known to destabilize mRNA and decrease receptor protein expression *in vitro* [76, 77]. GR-β, generated through an alternative splicing [78], is unable to bind ligand, is transcriptionally inactive, and exerts a dominant negative effect on transactivation by interfering with the binding of GR-α to the DNA [79, 80]. Honda et al. [81] reported GR-β specific mRNA expression in lymphocytes of 83 % of patients with steroid-resistant UC compared with only 9 % in responsive subjects and 10 % in healthy controls and patients with chronic active CD. This observation was confirmed in colonic biopsies of patients with UC: Significantly more GR-β-positive cells were seen in the resistant group than in the GC-sensitive and control group [82]. However, in IBD, GR-β is expressed 100–1,000 times less than GR-α, and this challenges its role in the genesis of steroid resistance in this disease. The role of *TthIIII*, ER22/23EK, and GR-9β has been investigated in association with the response to exogenous GCs. The combinations of the three polymorphisms were studied in 646 patients with multiple sclerosis treated with GCs. In this study, the haplotype consisting of *TthIIII*, ER22/23EK, and 9β-G was associated with GC resistance and with a more rapid disease progression. However, this seemed to result from the presence of ER22/23EK and not from the other two polymorphisms [83].

Two single nucleotide polymorphisms in the *NR3C1* gene, the N363S and *Bcl*I polymorphisms, have been, on the other hand, associated with an increased sensitivity to GCs. The N363S polymorphism, originally rs6195, currently listed in dbSNP as rs56149945, results in an asparagine (N) to serine (S) change in amino acid in codon 363. The N363S polymorphism may influence the interaction of the GR with coactivators and/or corepressors, one of the known functions of the N-terminal domain of this receptor [76]. Only few reports have studied the role of this polymorphism in the response to exogenous GCs. In 102 patients who underwent photorefractive keratectomy and received topical steroids as part of postoperative therapy, a significant correlation was found between N363S heterozygosity and ocular hypertension [84]. Furthermore, in 48 patients with Duchenne muscular dystrophy treated with prednisolone or deflazacort, the N363S carriers showed a trend toward a later age at loss of ambulation in comparison with noncarrier patients [85]. Only two studies to date have evaluated the role of this polymorphism in GC clinical response in IBD, but no relation was observed between the presence of this SNP and response to GCs both in pediatric and in adult patients [74, 75].

The *Bcl*I polymorphism (rs41423247) was initially described as a polymorphic restriction site inside intron 2, the nucleotide alteration was subsequently identified as a C>G substitution, 646 nucleotides downstream from exon 2 [86]. The molecular mechanism through which the *Bcl*I polymorphism exerts its effect is unknown. This polymorphism is associated with a clinical phenotype consistent with increased GC sensitivity in both heterozygous and homozygous carriers of the G allele. An association with unfavorable metabolic characteristics, such as increased body mass index and insulin resistance, has been also described [87]. The *Bcl*I SNP has been studied in 119 pediatric patients with IBD (64 with CD, 55 with UC). Patients were divided into two groups based on their response to GC treatment: GC dependence (45 patients) was defined by an initial response to prednisone with relapse on dose reduction, not allowing for steroid discontinuation, and GC responsiveness (67 patients) was defined as GC withdrawal without the need for steroids for at least 1 year. A significantly higher frequency of the *Bcl*I-mutated genotype was observed in the GC-responsive patients than in the GC-dependent group [74]. These results have been subsequently confirmed in a larger cohort of young patients with IBD [88] (Table 1).

miRNAs Involved in GR Regulation and Their Potential Role

Recently, noncoding miRNAs have emerged as important gene expression regulatory elements; understanding of the complex gene regulation may shed light on the causes of the variable responses to these hormones in patients with GC-sensitive or GC-resistant inflammatory and autoimmune diseases [89].

miRNAs are small (18–24 nucleotides) noncoding RNAs, which bind the 3′UTRs and the coding exons of their target genes and inhibit gene expression [90] either by messenger RNA (mRNA) cleavage (most common in plants) or by translational repression (most common in metazoan) [91, 92]. A single miRNA can regulate approximately 200 mRNAs, and each mRNA can be regulated by multiple miRNAs [93, 94]; overall, it is predicted that protein production for at least 20 % of all human genes is regulated by miRNAs [95, 96]. miRNAs suppress gene expression at the posttranscriptional level, and are fine-tuning regulators of diverse biological processes, including the development and function of the immune system, apoptosis, metabolism, and inflammation. Emerging data have implicated the deregulated expression of certain miRNA networks in the pathogenesis of

Table 1 Polymorphisms in the glucocorticoid receptor (GR) gene associated with altered glucocorticoid (GC) response in patients with inflammatory bowel disease (IBD) and other diseases

GR gene polymorphisms	Correlations with GC response in IBD or other diseases	References
TthIIII (rs10052957)	Correlation with elevated diurnal cortisol levels and reduced cortisol response to 1 mg dexamethasone (DEX), as well as lower insulin and cholesterol levels	[68]
	No correlation in haplotype with clinical response to GC in IBD patients	[72]
ER22/23EK (rs6189/rs6190)	Association with higher post-DEX cortisol levels and less cortisol suppression after a 1 mg DEX suppression test	[69]
	Correlation with a better metabolic and cardiovascular health profile and an increased survival	[70]
	In 119 pediatric patients with IBD, no association with GC response	[74]
	In adult IBD patients, no correlation with GC-resistant phenotype even when dividing patients into UC and CD	[75]
GR-9β (rs6198)	Association of the haplotype consisting of *TthIIII*, ER22/23EK, and GR-9β-G with GC resistance, and with a more rapid disease progression	[83]
N363S (rs6195)	Significant correlation with ocular hypertension in 102 patients who underwent photorefractive keratectomy and received topical steroids	[84]
	In 48 patients with Duchenne muscular dystrophy treated with prednisolone or deflazacort, correlation with a later age at loss of ambulation	[85]
	No correlation with response to GCs in pediatric IBD patients	[74]
	No correlation with response to GCs in adult IBD patients	[75]
BclI (rs41423247)	In 119 pediatric patients with IBD, association with GC response	[74]
	Unfavorable metabolic characteristics, such as increased body mass index and insulin resistance	[87]

autoimmune and inflammatory diseases, such as IBD, and it has been suggested that these small noncoding RNAs represent an important player in the complex interactions that result in IBD clinical features [97–100]. A number of studies have identified a specific differential expression of miRNAs in IBD and unique miRNA expression profiles for the different subtypes of IBDs and for evolutionary stages of the disease in colonoscopic biopsies [97, 101]. In particular, Zahm and colleagues [102] identified a number of miRNAs significantly increased in the serum of patients with pediatric CD in comparison with healthy subjects. In addition, Wu and colleagues demonstrated for the first time that peripheral blood miRNAs can distinguish active IBD subtypes from each other and healthy controls. They identified 10 miRNAs significantly increased and 1 miRNA significantly decreased in the peripheral blood of patients with active UC as compared with patients with CD, 12 miRNAs significantly increased and 1 miRNA significantly decreased in the blood of patients with active UC compared with healthy controls, and 5 miRNAs significantly increased and 2 miRNAs significantly decreased in the blood of patients with active CD compared with healthy controls [103]. Paraskevi and colleagues recently identified 11 miRNAs significantly increased in CD and 6 miRNAs increased in UC blood samples compared with healthy controls [104]: These results confirmed previous studies of IBD miRNA expression obtained in blood and/or tissue samples [98, 105].

In this context, the study of a possible correlation between tissue or blood miRNA expression and variability in GC response in pediatric patients with IBD could be a promising field of research. The investigation of miRNA expression as a pathogenetic or pharmacological biomarker in plasma, serum, or peripheral mononuclear cells instead of colonic tissues represents a semi-invasive diagnostic approach, easier to translate into clinical practice, particularly in a pediatric population. Indeed, an ideal biomarker must be easily accessible using noninvasive procedures, and this is especially true when the patients are children.

An important field of investigation concerns the role of miRNAs in the regulation of target genes, such as *NR3C1*. Computational studies showed that the 3′ UTR of the GR gene is predicted to contain numerous seed regions recognized by a variety of miRNAs [106].

Vreugdenhil and collaborators investigated the possible interaction between miRNAs and *NR3C1*, and they found that miR-18 and miR-124a bind GR mRNA and decrease GR activity in neuronal tissues, using a combination of *in silico* prediction of miRNA binding sites, miRNA overexpression studies, and mutagenesis of the GR 3′ UTR [107]. The overexpression of these miRNAs reduced GR protein levels and impaired the activation of the GC-responsive gene glucocorticoid-induced leucine zipper (*GILZ*) in neuronal cell cultures. In addition, these authors demonstrated by miRNA reporter assay that miR-124a is able to bind to the predicted seed region in the GR 3′UTR.

The role of miR-124 has been investigated in the regulation of GR expression in human T cells of patients with critical illness-related corticosteroid insufficiency. It was found that miR-124 specifically downregulated GR-α, and a slight increase of miR-124 and a reduction of GR-α were observed in patient T cells compared with healthy controls [108]. In addition, Tessel and colleagues [109] identified and characterized miR-130b as an important downregulator of GR in a GC-resistant multiple myeloma cell line: The overexpression of this miRNA was also associated with a decreased regulation of *GILZ*, a downstream GC-controlled gene (Table 2).

Table 2 Role of miRNA deregulation in inflammatory bowel disease (IBD) considering glucocorticoid receptor (GR) as target

Sample analyzed	Correlations	References
Patient colonoscopic pinch biopsies	miRNA expression changes during tissue inflammation, and patterns of miRNAs are intestine region-specific	[101]
Patient peripheral blood	miRNAs in peripheral blood can distinguish active IBD subtypes from each other and healthy controls	[103]
Patient serum	miRNA profiles significantly increased in the serum of patients with pediatric CD in comparison with healthy subjects	[102]
Patient blood samples	Pattern of 11 miRNAs significantly increased in CD and of 6 miRNAs in UC	[104]
In vitro neuronal cell cultures	miR-18 and miR-124a bind GR mRNA and decrease GR activity	[107]
Patient T cells	miR-124 in patients with critical illness-related corticosteroids insufficiency specifically downregulated GR-α	[108]
GC-resistant multiple myeloma cell line	miR-130b is an important downregulator of GR	[109]

CD Crohn's disease, *UC* ulcerative colitis

Conclusions

GCs have been used in the treatment of active IBD since the 1950s, and are still used to induce remission in pediatric IBD, but interindividual differences in their efficacy and several side effects have been reported. The main goal for clinicians is therefore to improve the efficacy and safety of these agents and, when possible, to reduce steroid exposure and use a nonsteroid option. This is particularly important in patients who do not respond and will suffer considerable steroid-dependent morbidity without any clinical gain. The molecular mechanisms involved in the variability in GC response are still not completely known, but advances in pharmacogenomics could contribute to the optimization and personalization of therapy. Pharmacogenomic studies represent a promising field of research that could increase our understanding of the pharmacology of steroids in IBDs and possibly in other diseases.

In conclusion, the identification of pharmacological, genetic, and epigenetic determinants associated with GC response in pediatric patients with IBD and the consequent personalization of therapy based on this information will result in higher quality, less toxicity, and a more rational employment of national health service resources.

References

1. Baldassano RN, Piccoli DA (1999) Inflammatory bowel disease in pediatric and adolescent patients. Gastroenterol Clin North Am 28(2):445–458
2. Hyams JS (1996) Crohn's disease in children. Pediatr Clin North Am 43(1):255–277
3. Michail S, Ramsy M, Soliman E (2012) Advances in inflammatory bowel diseases in children. Minerva Pediatr 64(3):257–270
4. Loftus EV Jr (2004) Clinical epidemiology of inflammatory bowel disease: incidence, prevalence, and environmental influences. Gastroenterology 126(6):1504–1517
5. Longobardi T, Jacobs P, Bernstein CN (2004) Utilization of health care resources by individuals with inflammatory bowel disease in the United States: a profile of time since diagnosis. Am J Gastroenterol 99(4):650–655
6. Carter MJ, Lobo AJ, Travis SP (2004) Guidelines for the management of inflammatory bowel disease in adults. Gut 53(Suppl 5):V1–V16
7. Ross SC, Strachan J, Russell RK, Wilson SL (2011) Psychosocial functioning and health-related quality of life in paediatric inflammatory bowel disease. J Pediatr Gastroenterol Nutr 53(5):480–488
8. Dretzke J, Edlin R, Round J, Connock M, Hulme C, Czeczot J, Fry-Smith A, McCabe C, Meads C (2011) A systematic review and economic evaluation of the use of tumour necrosis factor-alpha (TNF-alpha) inhibitors, adalimumab and infliximab, for Crohn's disease. Health Technol Assess (Winchester, England) 15(6):1–244
9. Friedman S (2004) General principles of medical therapy of inflammatory bowel disease. Gastroenterol Clin North Am 33(2):191–208, viii
10. Faubion WA Jr, Loftus EV Jr, Harmsen WS, Zinsmeister AR, Sandborn WJ (2001) The natural history of corticosteroid therapy for inflammatory bowel disease: a population-based study. Gastroenterology 121(2):255–260
11. Kansal S, Wagner J, Kirkwood CD, Catto-Smith AG (2013) Enteral nutrition in Crohn's disease: an underused therapy. Gastroenterol Res Pract 2013:482108
12. Markowitz J, Grancher K, Kohn N, Lesser M, Daum F (2000) A multicenter trial of 6-mercaptopurine and prednisone in children with newly diagnosed Crohn's disease. Gastroenterology 119(4):895–902
13. Hyams J, Markowitz J, Lerer T, Griffiths A, Mack D, Bousvaros A, Otley A, Evans J, Pfefferkorn M, Rosh J, Rothbaum R, Kugathasan S, Mezoff A, Wyllie R, Tolia V, delRosario JF, Moyer MS, Oliva-Hemker M, Leleiko N (2006) The natural history of corticosteroid therapy for ulcerative colitis in children. Clin Gastroenterol Hepatol 4(9):1118–1123
14. Markowitz J, Hyams J, Mack D, Leleiko N, Evans J, Kugathasan S, Pfefferkorn M, Mezoff A, Rosh J, Tolia V, Otley A, Griffiths A, Moyer MS, Oliva-Hemker M, Wyllie R, Rothbaum R, Bousvaros A, Del Rosario JF, Hale S, Lerer T (2006) Corticosteroid therapy in the age of infliximab: acute and 1-year outcomes in newly diagnosed children with Crohn's disease. Clin Gastroenterol Hepatol 4(9):1124–1129
15. Ruemmele FM, Veres G, Kolho KL, Griffiths A, Levine A, Escher JC, Amil Dias J, Barabino A, Braegger CP, Bronsky J, Buderus S, Martin-de-Carpi J, De Ridder L, Fagerberg UL, Hugot JP, Kierkus J, Kolacek S, Koletzko S, Lionetti P, Miele E, Navas Lopez VM, Paerregaard A, Russell RK, Serban DE, Shaoul R, Van Rheenen P, Veereman G, Weiss B, Wilson D, Dignass A, Eliakim A, Winter H, Turner D (2014) Consensus guidelines of ECCO/ESPGHAN on the medical management of pediatric Crohn's disease. J Crohns Colitis 8(10):1179–1207
16. Carvalho R, Hyams JS (2007) Diagnosis and management of inflammatory bowel disease in children. Semin Pediatr Surg 16(3):164–171
17. Thomsen OO, Cortot A, Jewell D, Wright JP, Winter T, Veloso FT, Vatn M, Persson T, Pettersson E (1998) A comparison of budesonide and mesalamine for active Crohn's disease. International Budesonide-Mesalamine Study Group. N Engl J Med 339(6):370–374

18. Wong SC, Macrae VE, McGrogan P, Ahmed SF (2006) The role of pro-inflammatory cytokines in inflammatory bowel disease growth retardation. J Pediatr Gastroenterol Nutr 43(2):144–155
19. Ballinger AB, Savage MO, Sanderson IR (2003) Delayed puberty associated with inflammatory bowel disease. Pediatr Res 53(2):205–210
20. Ezri J, Marques-Vidal P, Nydegger A (2012) Impact of disease and treatments on growth and puberty of pediatric patients with inflammatory bowel disease. Digestion 85(4):308–319
21. Wong SC, Catto-Smith AG, Zacharin M (2013) Pathological fractures in paediatric patients with inflammatory bowel disease. Eur J Pediatr 173(2):141–151
22. Vihinen MK, Kolho KL, Ashorn M, Verkasalo M, Raivio T (2008) Bone turnover and metabolism in paediatric patients with inflammatory bowel disease treated with systemic glucocorticoids. Eur J Endocrinol (European Federation of Endocrine Societies) 159(6):693–698
23. Weinstein RS, Jilka RL, Parfitt AM, Manolagas SC (1998) Inhibition of osteoblastogenesis and promotion of apoptosis of osteoblasts and osteocytes by glucocorticoids. Potential mechanisms of their deleterious effects on bone. J Clin Invest 102(2):274–282
24. Semeao EJ, Stallings VA, Peck SN, Piccoli DA (1997) Vertebral compression fractures in pediatric patients with Crohn's disease. Gastroenterology 112(5):1710–1713
25. Sidoroff M, Kolho KL (2014) Screening for adrenal suppression in children with inflammatory bowel disease discontinuing glucocorticoid therapy. BMC Gastroenterol 14:51
26. Desrame J, Sabate JM, Agher R, Bremont C, Gaudric M, Couturier D, Chaussade S (2002) Assessment of hypothalamic-pituitary-adrenal axis function after corticosteroid therapy in inflammatory bowel disease. Am J Gastroenterol 97(7):1785–1791
27. De Iudicibus S, Franca R, Martelossi S, Ventura A, Decorti G (2011) Molecular mechanism of glucocorticoid resistance in inflammatory bowel disease. World J Gastroenterol 17(9):1095–1108
28. Charmandari E, Kino T (2010) Chrousos syndrome: a seminal report, a phylogenetic enigma and the clinical implications of glucocorticoid signalling changes. Eur J Clin Invest 40(10):932–942. doi:10.1111/j.1365-2362.2010.02336.x
29. Charmandari E, Kino T, Chrousos GP (2013) Primary generalized familial and sporadic glucocorticoid resistance (Chrousos syndrome) and hypersensitivity. Endocr Dev 24:67–85
30. Beato M, Herrlich P, Schutz G (1995) Steroid hormone receptors: many actors in search of a plot. Cell 83(6):851–857
31. Davies P, Rushmere NK (1988) The structure and function of steroid receptors. Sci Prog 72(288 Pt 4):563–578
32. Theriault A, Boyd E, Harrap SB, Hollenberg SM, Connor JM (1989) Regional chromosomal assignment of the human glucocorticoid receptor gene to 5q31. Hum Genet 83(3):289–291
33. Baker AC, Green TL, Chew VW, Tung K, Amini A, Lim D, Cho K, Greenhalgh DG (2012) Enhanced steroid response of a human glucocorticoid receptor splice variant. Shock 38(1):11–17. doi:10.1097/SHK.0b013e318257c0c0
34. Lu NZ, Cidlowski JA (2004) The origin and functions of multiple human glucocorticoid receptor isoforms. Ann N Y Acad Sci 1024:102–123. doi:10.1196/annals.1321.008
35. Revollo JR, Cidlowski JA (2009) Mechanisms generating diversity in glucocorticoid receptor signaling. Ann N Y Acad Sci 1179:167–178. doi:10.1111/j.1749-6632.2009.04986.x
36. Zhou J, Cidlowski JA (2005) The human glucocorticoid receptor: one gene, multiple proteins and diverse responses. Steroids 70(5–7):407–417. doi:10.1016/j.steroids.2005.02.006
37. Oakley RH, Sar M, Cidlowski JA (1996) The human glucocorticoid receptor beta isoform. Expression, biochemical properties, and putative function. J Biol Chem 271(16):9550–9559
38. Wu I, Shin SC, Cao Y, Bender IK, Jafari N, Feng G, Lin S, Cidlowski JA, Schleimer RP, Lu NZ (2013) Selective glucocorticoid receptor translational isoforms reveal glucocorticoid-induced apoptotic transcriptomes. Cell Death Dis 4:e453. doi:10.1038/cddis.2012.193
39. Lu NZ, Cidlowski JA (2005) Translational regulatory mechanisms generate N-terminal glucocorticoid receptor isoforms with unique transcriptional target genes. Mol Cell 18(3):331–342. doi:10.1016/j.molcel.2005.03.025

40. Hutchison KA, Scherrer LC, Czar MJ, Ning Y, Sanchez ER, Leach KL, Deibel MR Jr, Pratt WB (1993) FK506 binding to the 56-kilodalton immunophilin (Hsp56) in the glucocorticoid receptor heterocomplex has no effect on receptor folding or function. Biochemistry 32(15):3953–3957
41. Pratt WB, Morishima Y, Murphy M, Harrell M (2006) Chaperoning of glucocorticoid receptors. Handb Exp Pharmacol 172:111–138
42. Gross KL, Lu NZ, Cidlowski JA (2009) Molecular mechanisms regulating glucocorticoid sensitivity and resistance. Mol Cell Endocrinol 300(1–2):7–16. doi:10.1016/j.mce.2008.10.001
43. Wikstrom AC (2003) Glucocorticoid action and novel mechanisms of steroid resistance: role of glucocorticoid receptor-interacting proteins for glucocorticoid responsiveness. J Endocrinol 178(3):331–337
44. Qian X, Zhu Y, Xu W, Lin Y (2001) Glucocorticoid receptor and heat shock protein 90 in peripheral blood mononuclear cells from asthmatics. Chin Med J (Engl) 114(10):1051–1054
45. Raddatz D, Middel P, Bockemuhl M, Benohr P, Wissmann C, Schworer H, Ramadori G (2004) Glucocorticoid receptor expression in inflammatory bowel disease: evidence for a mucosal down-regulation in steroid-unresponsive ulcerative colitis. Aliment Pharmacol Ther 19(1):47–61
46. Matysiak M, Makosa B, Walczak A, Selmaj K (2008) Patients with multiple sclerosis resisted to glucocorticoid therapy: abnormal expression of heat-shock protein 90 in glucocorticoid receptor complex. Mult Scler 14(7):919–926. doi:10.1177/1352458508090666
47. Damjanovic SS, Antic JA, Ilic BB, Cokic BB, Ivovic M, Ognjanovic SI, Isailovic TV, Popovic BM, Bozic IB, Tatic S, Matic G, Todorovic VN, Paunovic I (2012) Glucocorticoid receptor and molecular chaperones in the pathogenesis of adrenal incidentalomas: potential role of reduced sensitivity to glucocorticoids. Mol Med 18:1456–1465. doi:10.2119/molmed.2012.00261
48. Ouyang J, Chen P, Jiang T, Chen Y, Li J (2012) Nuclear HSP90 regulates the glucocorticoid responsiveness of PBMCs in patients with idiopathic nephrotic syndrome. Int Immunopharmacol 14(3):334–340. doi:10.1016/j.intimp.2012.08.012
49. Pemberton LF, Paschal BM (2005) Mechanisms of receptor-mediated nuclear import and nuclear export. Traffic 6(3):187–198. doi:10.1111/j.1600-0854.2005.00270.x
50. Almawi WY, Melemedjian OK (2002) Molecular mechanisms of glucocorticoid antiproliferative effects: antagonism of transcription factor activity by glucocorticoid receptor. J Leukoc Biol 71(1):9–15
51. Meijsing SH, Pufall MA, So AY, Bates DL, Chen L, Yamamoto KR (2009) DNA binding site sequence directs glucocorticoid receptor structure and activity. Science 324(5925):407–410. doi:10.1126/science.1164265
52. Nordeen SK, Suh BJ, Kuhnel B, Hutchison CA 3rd (1990) Structural determinants of a glucocorticoid receptor recognition element. Mol Endocrinol 4(12):1866–1873
53. De Bosscher K, Vanden Berghe W, Vermeulen L, Plaisance S, Boone E, Haegeman G (2000) Glucocorticoids repress NF-kappaB-driven genes by disturbing the interaction of p65 with the basal transcription machinery, irrespective of coactivator levels in the cell. Proc Natl Acad Sci U S A 97(8):3919–3924
54. Schacke H, Docke WD, Asadullah K (2002) Mechanisms involved in the side effects of glucocorticoids. Pharmacol Ther 96(1):23–43
55. Schacke H, Schottelius A, Docke WD, Strehlke P, Jaroch S, Schmees N, Rehwinkel H, Hennekes H, Asadullah K (2004) Dissociation of transactivation from transrepression by a selective glucocorticoid receptor agonist leads to separation of therapeutic effects from side effects. Proc Natl Acad Sci U S A 101(1):227–232. doi:10.1073/pnas.0300372101
56. Song IH, Gold R, Straub RH, Burmester GR, Buttgereit F (2005) New glucocorticoids on the horizon: repress, don't activate! J Rheumatol 32(7):1199–1207
57. Chen R, Burke TF, Cumberland JE, Brummet M, Beck LA, Casolaro V, Georas SN (2000) Glucocorticoids inhibit calcium- and calcineurin-dependent activation of the human IL-4 promoter. J Immunol 164(2):825–832
58. Yang-Yen HF, Chambard JC, Sun YL, Smeal T, Schmidt TJ, Drouin J, Karin M (1990) Transcriptional interference between c-Jun and the glucocorticoid receptor: mutual inhibition of DNA binding due to direct protein-protein interaction. Cell 62(6):1205–1215

59. Ray A, Prefontaine KE (1994) Physical association and functional antagonism between the p65 subunit of transcription factor NF-kappa B and the glucocorticoid receptor. Proc Natl Acad Sci U S A 91(2):752–756
60. Stocklin E, Wissler M, Gouilleux F, Groner B (1996) Functional interactions between Stat5 and the glucocorticoid receptor. Nature 383(6602):726–728. doi:10.1038/383726a0
61. Ing NH (2005) Steroid hormones regulate gene expression posttranscriptionally by altering the stabilities of messenger RNAs. Biol Reprod 72(6):1290–1296. doi:10.1095/biolreprod.105.040014
62. Croxtall JD, van Hal PT, Choudhury Q, Gilroy DW, Flower RJ (2002) Different glucocorticoids vary in their genomic and non-genomic mechanism of action in A549 cells. Br J Pharmacol 135(2):511–519. doi:10.1038/sj.bjp.0704474
63. Croxtall JD, Flower RJ (1992) Lipocortin 1 mediates dexamethasone-induced growth arrest of the A549 lung adenocarcinoma cell line. Proc Natl Acad Sci U S A 89(8):3571–3575
64. McConkey DJ, Nicotera P, Hartzell P, Bellomo G, Wyllie AH, Orrenius S (1989) Glucocorticoids activate a suicide process in thymocytes through an elevation of cytosolic Ca2+ concentration. Arch Biochem Biophys 269(1):365–370. doi:10.1016/0003-9861(89)90119-7
65. Cohen JJ, Duke RC (1984) Glucocorticoid activation of a calcium-dependent endonuclease in thymocyte nuclei leads to cell death. J Immunol 132(1):38–42
66. Ho GT, Chiam P, Drummond H, Loane J, Arnott ID, Satsangi J (2006) The efficacy of corticosteroid therapy in inflammatory bowel disease: analysis of a 5-year UK inception cohort. Aliment Pharmacol Ther 24(2):319–330
67. Hyams JS, Lerer T, Griffiths A, Pfefferkorn M, Kugathasan S, Evans J, Otley A, Carvalho R, Mack D, Bousvaros A, Rosh J, Mamula P, Kay M, Crandall W, Oliva-Hemker M, Keljo D, LeLeiko N, Markowitz J (2009) Long-term outcome of maintenance infliximab therapy in children with Crohn's disease. Inflamm Bowel Dis 15(6):816–822
68. van Rossum EF, Lamberts SW (2004) Polymorphisms in the glucocorticoid receptor gene and their associations with metabolic parameters and body composition. Recent Prog Horm Res 59:333–357
69. van Rossum EF, Koper JW, Huizenga NA, Uitterlinden AG, Janssen JA, Brinkmann AO, Grobbee DE, de Jong FH, van Duyn CM, Pols HA, Lamberts SW (2002) A polymorphism in the glucocorticoid receptor gene, which decreases sensitivity to glucocorticoids in vivo, is associated with low insulin and cholesterol levels. Diabetes 51(10):3128–3134
70. Manenschijn L, van den Akker EL, Lamberts SW, van Rossum EF (2009) Clinical features associated with glucocorticoid receptor polymorphisms. An overview. Ann N Y Acad Sci 1179:179–198
71. Detera-Wadleigh SD, Encio IJ, Rollins DY, Coffman D, Wiesch D (1991) A TthIII1 polymorphism on the 5′ flanking region of the glucocorticoid receptor gene (GRL). Nucleic Acids Res 19(8):1960. doi:10.1093/nar/19.8.1960-a
72. van Rossum EF, Roks PH, de Jong FH, Brinkmann AO, Pols HA, Koper JW, Lamberts SW (2004) Characterization of a promoter polymorphism in the glucocorticoid receptor gene and its relationship to three other polymorphisms. Clin Endocrinol (Oxf) 61(5):573–581
73. de Lange P, Koper JW, Huizenga NA, Brinkmann AO, de Jong FH, Karl M, Chrousos GP, Lamberts SW (1997) Differential hormone-dependent transcriptional activation and -repression by naturally occurring human glucocorticoid receptor variants. Mol Endocrinol (Baltimore, MD) 11(8):1156–1164
74. De Iudicibus S, Stocco G, Martelossi S, Drigo I, Norbedo S, Lionetti P, Pozzi E, Barabino A, Decorti G, Bartoli F, Ventura A (2007) Association of BclI polymorphism of the glucocorticoid receptor gene locus with response to glucocorticoids in inflammatory bowel disease. Gut 56(9):1319–1320
75. Maltese P, Palma L, Sfara C, de Rocco P, Latiano A, Palmieri O, Corritore G, Annese V, Magnani M (2012) Glucocorticoid resistance in Crohn's disease and ulcerative colitis: an association study investigating GR and FKBP5 gene polymorphisms. Pharmacogenomics J 12(5):432–438

76. Koper JW, van Rossum EF, van den Akker EL (2014) Glucocorticoid receptor polymorphisms and haplotypes and their expression in health and disease. Steroids 92C:62–73
77. Schaaf MJ, Cidlowski JA (2002) AUUUA motifs in the 3′UTR of human glucocorticoid receptor alpha and beta mRNA destabilize mRNA and decrease receptor protein expression. Steroids 67(7):627–636
78. Hagendorf A, Koper JW, de Jong FH, Brinkmann AO, Lamberts SW, Feelders RA (2005) Expression of the human glucocorticoid receptor splice variants alpha, beta, and P in peripheral blood mononuclear leukocytes in healthy controls and in patients with hyper- and hypocortisolism. J Clin Endocrinol Metab 90(11):6237–6243
79. Lewis-Tuffin LJ, Cidlowski JA (2006) The physiology of human glucocorticoid receptor beta (hGRbeta) and glucocorticoid resistance. Ann N Y Acad Sci 1069:1–9
80. Charmandari E, Chrousos GP, Ichijo T, Bhattacharyya N, Vottero A, Souvatzoglou E, Kino T (2005) The human glucocorticoid receptor (hGR) beta isoform suppresses the transcriptional activity of hGRalpha by interfering with formation of active coactivator complexes. Mol Endocrinol (Baltimore, MD) 19(1):52–64
81. Honda M, Orii F, Ayabe T, Imai S, Ashida T, Obara T, Kohgo Y (2000) Expression of glucocorticoid receptor beta in lymphocytes of patients with glucocorticoid-resistant ulcerative colitis. Gastroenterology 118(5):859–866. doi:10.1016/S0016-5085(00)70172-7
82. Fujishima S, Takeda H, Kawata S, Yamakawa M (2009) The relationship between the expression of the glucocorticoid receptor in biopsied colonic mucosa and the glucocorticoid responsiveness of ulcerative colitis patients. Clin Immunol (Orlando, FL) 133(2):208–217
83. van Winsen LL, Hooper-van Veen T, van Rossum EF, Polman CH, van den Berg TK, Koper JW, Uitdehaag BM (2005) The impact of glucocorticoid receptor gene polymorphisms on glucocorticoid sensitivity is outweighted in patients with multiple sclerosis. J Neuroimmunol 167(1–2):150–156
84. Szabo V, Borgulya G, Filkorn T, Majnik J, Banyasz I, Nagy ZZ (2007) The variant N363S of glucocorticoid receptor in steroid-induced ocular hypertension in Hungarian patients treated with photorefractive keratectomy. Mol Vis 13:659–666
85. Bonifati DM, Witchel SF, Ermani M, Hoffman EP, Angelini C, Pegoraro E (2006) The glucocorticoid receptor N363S polymorphism and steroid response in Duchenne dystrophy. J Neurol Neurosurg Psychiatry 77(10):1177–1179. doi:10.1136/jnnp.2005.078345
86. van Rossum EF, Koper JW, van den Beld AW, Uitterlinden AG, Arp P, Ester W, Janssen JA, Brinkmann AO, de Jong FH, Grobbee DE, Pols HA, Lamberts SW (2003) Identification of the BclI polymorphism in the glucocorticoid receptor gene: association with sensitivity to glucocorticoids in vivo and body mass index. Clin Endocrinol (Oxf) 59(5):585–592
87. Di Blasio AM, van Rossum EF, Maestrini S, Berselli ME, Tagliaferri M, Podesta F, Koper JW, Liuzzi A, Lamberts SW (2003) The relation between two polymorphisms in the glucocorticoid receptor gene and body mass index, blood pressure and cholesterol in obese patients. Clin Endocrinol (Oxf) 59(1):68–74
88. De Iudicibus S, Stocco G, Martelossi S, Londero M, Ebner E, Pontillo A, Lionetti P, Barabino A, Bartoli F, Ventura A, Decorti G (2010) Genetic predictors of glucocorticoid response in pediatric patients with inflammatory bowel diseases. J Clin Gastroenterol 45(1):e1–e7. doi:10.1097/MCG.0b013e3181e8ae93
89. Lane SJ, Adcock IM, Richards D, Hawrylowicz C, Barnes PJ, Lee TH (1998) Corticosteroid-resistant bronchial asthma is associated with increased c-fos expression in monocytes and T lymphocytes. J Clin Invest 102(12):2156–2164
90. Guo H, Ingolia NT, Weissman JS, Bartel DP (2010) Mammalian microRNAs predominantly act to decrease target mRNA levels. Nature 466(7308):835–840. doi:10.1038/nature09267
91. Rigoutsos I (2009) New tricks for animal microRNAS: targeting of amino acid coding regions at conserved and nonconserved sites. Cancer Res 69(8):3245–3248. doi:10.1158/0008-5472.CAN-09-0352
92. Bartel DP (2004) MicroRNAs: genomics, biogenesis, mechanism, and function. Cell 116(2):281–297

93. Lewis BP, Shih IH, Jones-Rhoades MW, Bartel DP, Burge CB (2003) Prediction of mammalian microRNA targets. Cell 115(7):787–798
94. Lewis BP, Burge CB, Bartel DP (2005) Conserved seed pairing, often flanked by adenosines, indicates that thousands of human genes are microRNA targets. Cell 120(1):15–20. doi:10.1016/j.cell.2004.12.035
95. Friedman Y, Balaga O, Linial M (2013) Working together: combinatorial regulation by microRNAs. Adv Exp Med Biol 774:317–337. doi:10.1007/978-94-007-5590-1_16
96. Singh TR, Gupta A, Suravajhala P (2013) Challenges in the miRNA research. Int J Bioinform Res Appl 9(6):576–583. doi:10.1504/IJBRA.2013.056620
97. Iborra M, Bernuzzi F, Invernizzi P, Danese S (2012) MicroRNAs in autoimmunity and inflammatory bowel disease: crucial regulators in immune response. Autoimmun Rev 11(5):305–314
98. Archanioti P, Gazouli M, Theodoropoulos G, Vaiopoulou A, Nikiteas N (2011) Micro-RNAs as regulators and possible diagnostic bio-markers in inflammatory bowel disease. J Crohns Colitis 5(6):520–524. doi:10.1016/j.crohns.2011.05.007
99. Coskun M, Bjerrum JT, Seidelin JB, Nielsen OH (2012) MicroRNAs in inflammatory bowel disease–pathogenesis, diagnostics and therapeutics. World J Gastroenterol 18(34):4629–4634. doi:10.3748/wjg.v18.i34.4629
100. Dalal SR, Kwon JH (2010) The role of microRNA in inflammatory bowel disease. Gastroenterol Hepatol (N Y) 6(11):714–722
101. Wu F, Zhang S, Dassopoulos T, Harris ML, Bayless TM, Meltzer SJ, Brant SR, Kwon JH (2010) Identification of microRNAs associated with ileal and colonic Crohn's disease. Inflamm Bowel Dis 16(10):1729–1738
102. Zahm AM, Thayu M, Hand NJ, Horner A, Leonard MB, Friedman JR (2011) Circulating microRNA is a biomarker of pediatric Crohn disease. J Pediatr Gastroenterol Nutr 53(1):26–33
103. Wu F, Guo NJ, Tian H, Marohn M, Gearhart S, Bayless TM, Brant SR, Kwon JH (2011) Peripheral blood microRNAs distinguish active ulcerative colitis and Crohn's disease. Inflamm Bowel Dis 17(1):241–250
104. Paraskevi A, Theodoropoulos G, Papaconstantinou I, Mantzaris G, Nikiteas N, Gazouli M (2012) Circulating microRNA in inflammatory bowel disease. J Crohns Colitis 6(9):900–904
105. Pekow JR, Kwon JH (2012) MicroRNAs in inflammatory bowel disease. Inflamm Bowel Dis 18(1):187–193
106. Kertesz M, Iovino N, Unnerstall U, Gaul U, Segal E (2007) The role of site accessibility in microRNA target recognition. Nat Genet 39(10):1278–1284. doi:10.1038/ng2135
107. Vreugdenhil E, Verissimo CS, Mariman R, Kamphorst JT, Barbosa JS, Zweers T, Champagne DL, Schouten T, Meijer OC, de Kloet ER, Fitzsimons CP (2009) MicroRNA 18 and 124a down-regulate the glucocorticoid receptor: implications for glucocorticoid responsiveness in the brain. Endocrinology 150(5):2220–2228. doi:10.1210/en.2008-1335
108. Ledderose C, Mohnle P, Limbeck E, Schutz S, Weis F, Rink J, Briegel J, Kreth S (2012) Corticosteroid resistance in sepsis is influenced by microRNA-124–induced downregulation of glucocorticoid receptor-alpha. Crit Care Med 40(10):2745–2753. doi:10.1097/CCM.0b013e31825b8ebc
109. Tessel MA, Benham AL, Krett NL, Rosen ST, Gunaratne PH (2011) Role for microRNAs in regulating glucocorticoid response and resistance in multiple myeloma. Horm Cancer 2(3):182–189. doi:10.1007/s12672-011-0072-8

Corticosteroids in Pediatric Dermatology

Stefano Cambiaghi and Carlo Gelmetti

Introduction

Ever since their introduction, corticosteroids have been popular drugs in dermatology; in skin disorders they are prescribed topically or systemically. Intralesional administration is also possible but is a rare occurrence in childhood. Corticosteroids are commonly used in dermatological practice in both children and adults for their anti-inflammatory, immunosuppressive, and antiproliferative action. In general, treatment with this class of drugs should be of adequate potency and conveniently tapered, avoiding abrupt interruption [1].

Systemic Corticosteroids

Systemic corticosteroids are among the drugs most widely used by dermatologists for a wide variety of cutaneous diseases [2]. Although their use in pediatric dermatology patients is limited, systemic corticosteroids are required in the management of some skin disorders because of their severity or because of their intrinsic nature or extracutaneous involvement.

In pediatric dermatology, systemic corticosteroids remain the cornerstone treatment for autoimmune blistering diseases, including pemphigus and pemphigoid, and for connective tissue disorders, including lupus erythematosus and dermatomyositis. In addition, systemic corticosteroids can be used in some forms of vasculitis, in acute allergic reactions, and in severe forms of erythema multiforme and erythema nodosum (see Table 1). Severe flare-ups of atopic dermatitis often require

S. Cambiaghi (✉) • C. Gelmetti
Department of Pathophysiology and Transplantation, University of Milan, Fondazione IRCCS Ca' Granda "Ospedale Maggiore Policlinico", Milan, Via Pace 9, 20122 Milan, Italy
e-mail: stefano.cambiaghi@fastwebnet.it

R. Cimaz (ed.), *Systemic Corticosteroids for Inflammatory Disorders in Pediatrics*, DOI 10.1007/978-3-319-16056-6_10

Table 1 Indications for systemic corticosteroid treatment in pediatric dermatology

Connective tissue disorders
Systemic lupus erythematosus
Dermatomyositis
Scleroderma
Bullous disorders
Linear immunoglobulin A bullous dermatosis
Bullous pemphigoid
Pemphigus vulgaris
Dermatitis herpetiformis
Erythema multiforme
Vasculitis
Polyarteritis nodosa
Henoch–Schönlein purpura
Granulomatous vasculitides
Behçet's disease
Neutrophilic disorders
Pyoderma gangrenosum
Sweet's syndrome
Inflammatory skin disorders
Atopic dermatitis (flares)
Irritant and allergic contact dermatitis
Urticaria/angioedema (acute)
Erythroderma (various underlying cause)
Miscellaneous disorders
Infantile hemangiomas
Alopecia areata
Lichen planus
Drug reactions
Erythema nodosum

short courses of systemic corticosteroids, although these drugs are not recommended for routine long-term treatment [3].

The daily dose of steroids depends on the severity of the disease and on the clinical parameters of the patient. A typical initial dose for most moderate to severe dermatologic conditions is 1.0 mg/kg of prednisone or prednisone-equivalent per day [4]. Short courses (less than 4 weeks) of corticosteroid therapy are usually safe and effective in treating acute skin diseases. In long-term treatments, adjuvant or steroid-sparing agents such as other immunosuppressive drugs, antimalarials, and sulfones are often used in an attempt to reduce the dose of corticosteroids required to control the disease. Very short courses (2–3 weeks or less) of corticosteroids do not necessitate tapering, although most clinicians do not stop the treatment abruptly so as to eliminate the risk of disease recurrence and of steroid withdrawal symptoms.

In pediatric dermatology, the most common route of systemic administration is the oral route, with a steroid molecule of intermediate anti-inflammatory potency, such as prednisone, usually given in an early morning single dose [5]. General recommendations for corticosteroid use are valid in dermatological practice as well. The therapeutic dosage of systemic corticosteroids used in skin disorders, most often ranging from 0.5 to 1.5 mg/kg/day, may cause suppression of the hypothalamic–pituitary–adrenal axis and growth suppression in the long-term treatment of pediatric patients. Because long-acting agents such as dexamethasone are highly effective in suppression of the hypothalamic–pituitary–adrenal axis, and because hydrocortisone and cortisone acetate are too short-acting for a lasting therapeutic effect, most dermatologists are likely to use prednisone or methylprednisolone [6]. While the latter is an excellent choice for minimizing the mineralocorticoid effects, prednisone is cheap, widely available, and marketed in many dosage forms.

Systemic corticosteroid therapy produces cutaneous side effects similar to those of Cushing's syndrome, which are well known to dermatologists, including striae distensae, purpura, telangiectasia, atrophy, steroid acne, hirsutism, alopecia, hyperpigmentation, and wound healing impairment. Of these, striae distensae are permanent, while the others may be reversible.

In acute self-limited steroid-sensitive skin disorders, such as severe contact dermatitis, a short (1–2 weeks) course of oral prednisone is usually started and rapidly tapered. In acute allergic or anaphylactic reactions, for example, following insect bites or drug reactions, hydrocortisone is usually given intravenously accompanied by antihistamines [7].

Autoimmune bullous diseases such as pemphigus, pemphigoid, dermatitis herpetiformis, and linear immunoglobulin A dermatitis are rare in children but they require vigorous corticosteroid therapy when diagnosed [8]. Childhood bullous pemphigoid is usually responsive to moderate prednisone doses (0.5–1 mg/kg/day), while pemphigus vulgaris is more difficult to control and requires larger doses to achieve remission. The use of corticosteroid-sparing agents is often necessary to reduce corticosteroid side effects in the treatment of pemphigus vulgaris. Dapsone is possibly a better therapeutic option for dermatitis herpetiformis and linear immunoglobulin A dermatitis, but concomitant use of corticosteroids is required, at least initially, to achieve better results.

A wide spectrum of therapeutic agents with anti-inflammatory and immunosuppressive action are available in the treatment of juvenile-onset systemic lupus erythematosus. Among these, low doses of systemic corticosteroids are useful in controlling minor manifestations of the disease, while higher doses are still used to manage major manifestations that can endanger the patient's life [9].

Aggressive management with high-dose oral systemic corticosteroids, with or without other drugs, is the traditional treatment for juvenile dermatomyositis. Aggressive treatment directed at achieving a rapid and complete control of muscle inflammation is highly successful in minimizing the long-term sequelae of the disorder, including calcinosis. High oral doses of prednisone (1.5–2 mg/kg daily) or pulse intravenous methylprednisone therapy (30 mg/kg) are used [10]. Pulse intravenous corticosteroid therapy is usually preferred to maintain efficacy while lowering the side effects [11], although this treatment may lead to muscle strength deterioration and no long-term changes in the outcome [12]. Some authors suggest that early intervention with additional immunomodulatory agents allows for a faster recovery, with less medication and fewer disease sequelae [13].

Pulsed intravenous corticosteroid therapy is often used in connective tissue disorders (dermatomyositis, scleroderma) allowing for a shorter course of therapy with fewer long-term side effects. Usually, a single high daily dose of methylprednisolone is given intravenously over 2 h 1–5 (but usually 3) consecutive days per month. Children seem to tolerate this regimen exceedingly well. Sudden death of cardiac arrest, possibly due to a sudden electrolyte shift, has been described in adults, so that appropriate cardiologic monitoring is mandatory during treatment.

High-dose intravenous methylprednisolone on 3 consecutive days given monthly and accompanied by a low weekly dose of methotrexate (0.3–0.6 mg/kg) is standard treatment for children with localized severe forms of cutaneous scleroderma [14]. Although consensus on specific regimens is lacking [15], the dose of the drug in the literature is 30 mg/kg/day (not exceeding 500 mg) for 3 days monthly for 3 months. This regimen appears to be effective and is generally well tolerated by children [16]. Problems of renal, cardiac, and endocrine nature must be carefully assessed before starting the procedure, while blood pressure, urinalysis, full blood count, renal and liver function, and electrolytes should be monitored during treatment.

Systemic steroids have represented the mainstay of treatment for problematic infantile hemangiomas for many years thanks to their well-known antiproliferative and antiangiogenic properties [17]. Usually, a prednisone-equivalent daily dose of 1–3 mg/kg is administered for weeks to months in the proliferating phase of the hemangioma [18]. Although systemic propranolol has currently become the first-line treatment for infantile hemangiomas worldwide, systemic steroids are still used if β-blockers are contraindicated.

Alopecia areata is a common disorder affecting the scalp and body hair. It may occur at any age, but usually appears before the age of 20 years. Although the exact etiology of the disorder is still unclear, corticosteroids are widely used in both topical and systemic administration. Topical clobetasol propionate has been proven effective in inducing hair regrowth as a result of a local effect [19]. The usefulness of systemic corticosteroids as a therapeutic modality for severe forms of alopecia areata remains a matter of debate. Oral daily prednisone intake of 0.5–1 mg/kg/day may induce satisfactory regrowth in 40 % of patients, but this result is often not maintained after treatment. In children with widespread alopecia areata, intravenous methylprednisolone pulses on 3 consecutive days in 1-month intervals [20] or single high oral doses of prednisolone in 1-month intervals [21] have also been used. Short disease duration, younger age at onset, and multifocal as opposed to severe diffuse alopecia are positive prognostic factors in alopecia areata. Unfortunately, in patients with alopecia totalis and universalis, even pulse therapy is often disappointing.

Vitiligo is a common chronic and often progressive disorder of possible autoimmune origin causing disfiguring depigmentation in children and adults.

Systemic corticosteroids have been used to arrest disease progression and to induce repigmentation. The effectiveness of low-dose oral corticosteroids in preventing the progression of the disease has been reported and represents a therapeutic option in patients difficult to treat, with spreading disease, or not responding to other treatments (e.g., topical corticosteroids and photochemotherapy) [22]. Treatment schedules include the use of an oral mini-pulse with 2.5, 5, or 10 mg of betamethasone or dexamethasone on 2 consecutive days per week after breakfast [23, 24]. Although children have been included in some of the published studies, conclusions on long-term efficacy are lacking, especially in the pediatric population.

In a subset of patients affected by severe or recalcitrant psoriasis, including arthropathic, pustular, and erythrodermic forms, systemic treatment is needed. Although systemic steroids are rapidly effective in psoriasis at the beginning of treatment, tachyphylaxis also ensues quickly. Worsening with possible induction of severe, often generalized, pustular psoriasis may be observed as a treatment outcome. Hence, systemic steroids are not an option in these patients, who should receive other treatment (e.g., phototherapy, acitretin, methotrexate, cyclosporine, or tumor necrosis factor-α inhibitors) [25].

Intramuscular administration of corticosteroids for dermatological disorders is seldom required in pediatric practice. Advantages include close physician control over therapy, guaranteed compliance, and assured absorption [5]. Sterile abscesses, hypopigmentation, and local atrophy at the injection site are well-known side effects of both intramuscular and intralesional corticosteroid therapy.

Intramuscular injection of corticosteroids remains the most common cause of postinjectional atrophy. Antibiotics, insulin, human growth hormone, and vasopressin are other possible causative drugs. Steroids act by increasing lipolysis while inhibiting lipogenesis and fibroblast activity. Reports on this topic are mainly focused on triamcinolone and on steroids in poorly soluble forms, such as triamcinolone acetonide. The occurrence of atrophy is related to the power, the quantity, the concentration, and the solubility of the drug as well as to the anatomical level of the injection. The deeper the injection, the lower the atrophy, which is likely to occur when the needle fails to reach the muscular tissue. Subcutaneous atrophy after corticosteroid injection is usually self-healing in the pediatric patient, although it may take many months for the damaged skin to go back to normal.

The intralesional injection of corticosteroids, as mentioned, is of limited use in pediatric patients. Main applications of intralesional corticosteroids include nail lichen, keloids, and focal persistent areas of alopecia areata. Local pain and the risk of atrophy must be taken into consideration. Corticosteroids should not be injected more often than every 4–6 weeks to avoid severe atrophy at the injection site. Especially in the case of *depot* forms of corticosteroids, it should be assumed that the total dose of the drug is absorbed systemically and may have systemic effect including adrenal suppression.

Topical Corticosteroids

Treatment with topical corticosteroids (TCS) remains pivotal in the management of many skin diseases requiring anti-inflammatory effect, but their efficacy depends on three fundamental principles: sufficient strength, sufficient dosage, and correct application. In addition, it should be remembered that topical treatment should always be applied after the skin has been cleansed.

As the skin is an external organ, the role of systemic corticosteroid therapy is limited by the possibility of direct application of the drug on the skin surface. Thus, in pediatric dermatology a number of disorders may be managed by topical preparations directly exerting a local action in the damaged area with few or no systemic side effects. The use of topical corticosteroid preparations has become a common treatment in numerous settings, and their anti-inflammatory and antiproliferative action is being used in everyday practice in pediatric dermatology to control different skin diseases, of which atopic dermatitis remains by far the most common [26]. Both chronic, such as atopic dermatitis, and mild to moderate acute inflammatory skin conditions, such as contact dermatitis, of both allergic and irritative origin, insect bites, psoriasis, lichen planus, lichen sclerosus and atrophicus, and alopecia areata, are usually managed with TCS [3].

However, TCS have a nonspecific effect or may be unable to modify the natural course of the skin disorder. This can result in recurrence of the skin disease at the end of treatment or occasionally in severe flaring-up: The *rebound phenomenon* may be observed after systemic or topical treatment. Moreover, corticosteroids are so effective in controlling the signs and symptoms of inflammatory skin disorders that both patients and doctors may overlook the importance of other necessary measures, such as avoiding allergens in contact allergic dermatitis, performing skin scraping to exclude fungal infections, etc.

TCS of different strength are available. As a general rule, the potency of the corticosteroid to be prescribed and the duration of the topical treatment must be weighed against the severity and the extension of the dermatitis, the anatomical area to be treated, and the patient's age. In potency ranking, clobetasol propionate and halcinonide are at the top, while hydrocortisone is at the bottom [1, 27]. The power of the topical corticosteroid depends on the molecule[1] and on its concentration in the marketed preparation. A wide range of different molecules are available in a variety of formulations. TCS are classified into potency groups that should be known to prescribers: groups I (mild), II (moderate), III (potent), and IV (very potent). It should be noted that the American system is reversed and divided into seven classes, ranging from class I (super potent) to class VII (low potency). Usually, the acute phases of atopic dermatitis are controlled with one to two applications of a potent TCS cream over the day (Table 2). Lipid-soluble corticosteroids such as

---

[1]Potency is an intrinsic property of the drug and not the same thing as concentration. Of note: potency can be altered by drug concentration and formulation (nature of vehicle used). Therefore, in daily practice, it is sometimes incorrectly thought that topical steroid drug concentration relates to potency.

Table 2 Examples of topical corticosteroids ranking

Topical corticosteroids ranking in the EU

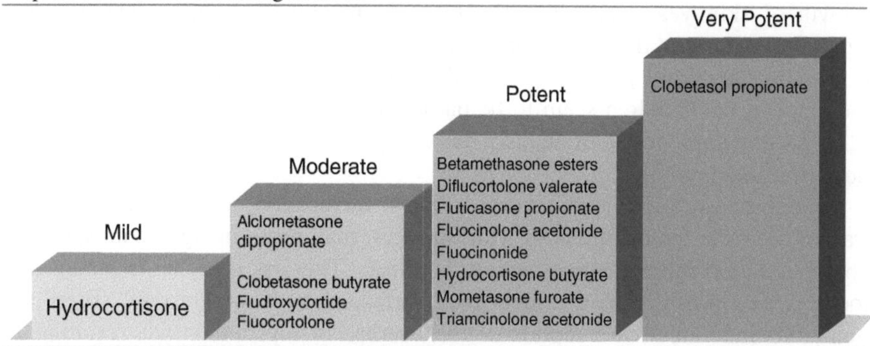

Topical corticosteroids ranking in the USA

Class	*Potency*	*Example*	*Formulation*
Class I	Ultra high	Clobetasol propionate 0.05 %	All formulations
Class II	High	Betamethasone dipropionate 0.05 %	Ointment
Class III	Medium to high	Betamethasone dipropionate 0.05 %	Cream
Class IV and V	Medium	Mometasone furoate 0.1 %	All formulations
		Hydrocortisone butyrate 0.1 %	Ointment
Class VI	Low	Hydrocortisone butyrate 0.1 %	Cream
		Alclometasone dipropionate 0.05 %	All formulations
Class VII	Least potent	Hydrocortisone 1 and 2.5 %	All formulations

www.topicalsteroids.co.uk

fluocinolone acetonide tend to be clinically more potent, because they penetrate the skin more rapidly and efficaciously. Hydrocortisone on the other hand is relatively lipid insoluble. Not only the molecule but also its vehicle is of paramount importance in influencing the absorption and the potency of the drug. Creams, ointments, gel, and lotions penetrate the skin differently; for example, ointments are usually more effective than creams, which in turn are more effective than lotions. The efficacy of ointments is useful in treating chronic or hyperkeratotic lesions or in palmoplantar dermatoses. On the other hand, ointments are greasy and occlusive, and their use may be unsuitable in humid environments, on hair-bearing skin, or in body flexures. Creams are more patient-friendly and are preferred in acute and subacute dermatoses and on moist skin. Lotions are suitable for application on hair-bearing areas, but they often have an alcoholic vehicle that can burn or sting when applied on damaged skin. However, the distinction between these vehicles is becoming less clear as new topical delivery systems are developed.

Corticosteroids tend to accumulate in the stratum corneum when applied, with subsequent progressive release in the deeper layers of the skin. This *reservoir effect* may explain why once-daily application of TCS is usually enough in most dermatoses. However, when the stratum corneum is absent, as can occur in some inflammatory conditions, the reservoir effect may be lost and a higher number of daily applications is justified.

Local side effects of TCS application include skin atrophy with epidermal thinning, miliaria, telangiectasia, hypopigmentation, increased hair growth, and overgrowth of skin yeasts and bacteria, possibly resulting in impetiginization and candidiasis. Perioral dermatitis, acne flares, and rosacea may follow TCS application on the face, while granuloma gluteale infantum may follow TCS application on the diaper area. Children seem to be particularly susceptible to these side effects [27]. A dermatophytosis erroneously treated by TCS may become difficult to diagnose (tinea incognito).

Moreover, excessive application of topical medication, as in the case of protracted use or in the treatment of wide surfaces, may result in significant systemic absorption with subsequent systemic side effects. This risk is higher in infants and toddlers, because they have a high body surface-to-body weight ratio. There are numerous individual case reports of the overuse of topical steroids resulting in growth suppression, adrenal failure, and Cushing's syndrome. Most of these reports involve the use of potent fluorinated topical corticosteroids on inflamed skin. Percutaneous absorption is influenced by the thickness of the stratum corneum and by its lipid composition. Clinicians should be aware that absorption is very high in skin areas such as the eyelids, the parotid region, the scrotum, and the vulva [28]. In addition, some skin disorders (e.g., erythroderma, Netherton syndrome) may predispose the child to a higher absorption of topical drugs through the skin.

Potent or superpotent TCS should be avoided in children or used for a limited amount of time. Occlusive medications increase TCS potency by enhancing their epidermal concentration and absorption. They should be avoided in children to prevent significant skin atrophy. Skinfold areas provide natural occlusion, especially in infants, so that low-potency preparations are more suitable there. For the same reason, topical corticosteroids should not be routinely used in the diaper area of infants. On the face, their application should be avoided if possible, but if needed, corticosteroids of low potency should be used.

In atopic dermatitis aggressive topical corticosteroid therapy is crucial in the management of flares. The golden rule for TCS prescription in atopic dermatitis, "better strong than long, but treat as weak as effective," may be true and useful in almost every skin disorder. To date, TCS remain the first-line topical anti-inflammatory option in atopic dermatitis. They should be applied on inflammatory skin according to the needs of the patient (pruritus, sleeplessness, new flare). Parents and patients should be trained to apply the drug on the inflamed skin only, and to gradually reduce its application as soon as a satisfactory result has been achieved. To avoid tachyphylaxis, twice-daily application should not last longer than 1 week, with subsequent gradual tapering. Dose tapering should be gradual to avoid withdrawal rebound; tapering strategies consist in using a less potent corticosteroid on a daily basis, or keeping a more potent one while reducing the frequency of application (intermittent regimen). Recently twice weekly proactive[2] topical

[2] Proactive therapy is defined as long-term, low-dose, intermittent application of anti-inflammatory treatment to previously affected skin, together with daily application of emollients to unaffected areas. This "minimal therapy for minimal eczema" regimen is continued after clearance of the visible eczema at a low frequency – usually twice weekly.

treatment with corticosteroids (but also with topical calcineurin inhibitors such as tacrolimus or pimecrolimus) has proven effective in reducing the number of atopic dermatitis flares and the side effects of topical steroid use with a good cost–effectiveness ratio [29].

Some patients with very inflamed lesions do not tolerate standard topical application, and may first be treated with the so-called wet wrap(s) technique (WWT) until the oozing stops [30]. WWT is usually performed using a topical corticosteroid based-cream and a double layer of cotton bandages, with a moist first layer and a dry second layer. The topical medication can be applied as usual on the skin or previously diluted in lukewarm water in which the first layer is moistened. The use of WWT for up to 14 days (usually 2–3 days) is a safe treatment for severe and/or refractory atopic dermatitis and is almost always characterized by a dramatic improvement in the disease. What is normally overlooked (even by doctors) is that topical therapy is time consuming (WWT, of course, is even more time consuming), and techniques such as WWT have to be practically illustrated by doctors or nurses, at least for the first application.

TCS are often marketed in combination with other active compounds, such as topical antibiotics or antifungal agents. Dermatologists are not usually fond of these combinations, which are often used in the absence of a specific diagnosis, but they have some usefulness when an infection is thought to coexist with the inflammatory condition. The possibility that both the active and inactive ingredients contained in the marketed TCS preparation may cause an allergic reaction must be considered. Also, the possible occurrence of an allergic contact dermatitis to the corticosteroid itself is a rare but known phenomenon [31]. Although unusual, these events should be suspected if TCS treatment for a skin disorder that is usually responsive to corticosteroids fails. In this case, patch testing may provide the clue to the diagnosis.

Finally, the occurrence of *corticophobia*, the fear among patients and their parents of using topical corticosteroids, is a complex phenomenon in developed countries. Corticophobia should always be assessed before corticosteroid prescription in order to avoid low compliance to the treatment [32].

References

1. Barnetson RS, White AD (1992) The use of corticosteroids in dermatological practice. Med J Aust 156:428–431
2. Williams LC, Nesbitt LT (2001) Update on systemic glucocorticosteroids in dermatology. Dermatol Clin 19:63–77
3. Harper J, Oranje A, Prose N (2006) Textbook of pediatric dermatology, 2nd edn. Blackwell Publishing Ltd, Oxford
4. Byekova YA, Hughey LC, Elewski BE (2011) Systemic drugs in patients with skin diseases. G Ital Dermatol Venereol 146:397–424
5. Nesbitt LT Jr (1995) Minimizing complications from systemic glucocorticosteroids use. Dermatol Clin 13:925–939
6. Lucky AW (1984) Principles of the use of glucocorticosteroids in the growing child. Pediatr Dermatol 3:226–235

7. Burns T, Breathnach S, Cox N, Griffiths C (2010) Rook's textbook of dermatology, 8th edn. Wiley-Blackwell Publishing, Oxford
8. Fritz KA, Weston WL (1984) Systemic glucocorticosteroid therapy of skin disease in children. Pediatr Dermatol 1:236–245
9. Carreno L, Lopez-Longo FJ, Gonzalez CM, Monteagudo I (2002) Treatment options for juvenile-onset systemic lupus erythematosus. Pediatr Drugs 4:241–256
10. Fisler RE, Liang MG, Fuhlbrigge RC, Yalcndag A, Sundel RP (2002) Aggressive management of juvenile dermatomyositis results in improved outcome and decreased incidence of calcinosis. J Am Acad Dermatol 47:505–511
11. Paller AS (1996) The use of pulse corticosteroid therapy for juvenile dermatomyositis. Pediatr Dermatol 13:347–348
12. Lang B, Dooley J (1996) Failure of pulse intravenous methylprednisolone treatment in juvenile dermatomyositis. J Pediatr 128:429–432
13. Reed AM, Lopez M (2002) Juvenile dermatomyositis: recognition and treatment. Pediatr Drugs 4:315–321
14. Weibel L, Sampaio MC, Visentin MT, Howell KJ, Woo P, Harper JI (2006) Evaluation of methotrexate and corticosteroids for the treatment of localized scleroderma (morphoea) in children. Br J Dermatol 155:1013–1020
15. Li SC, Feldman BM, Higgins GC, Haines KA, Punaro MG, O'Neil KM (2010) Treatment of pediatric localized scleroderma: results of a survey of North American pediatric rheumatologists. J Rheumatol 37:175–181
16. Uziel Y, Feldman BM, Krafchik BR, Yeung RS, Laxer RM (2000) Methotrexate and corticosteroid therapy for pediatric localized scleroderma. J Pediatr 136:91–95
17. Bennett ML, Fleischer AB Jr, Chamlin SL, Frieden IJ (2001) Oral corticosteroid use is effective for cutaneous hemangiomas: an evidence-based evaluation. Arch Dermatol 137:1208–1213
18. Pope E, Krafchik BR, Macarthur C, Stempak D, Stephens D, Weinstein M, Ho N, Baruchel S (2007) Oral versus high-dose pulse corticosteroids for problematic infantile hemangiomas: a randomized, controlled trial. Pediatrics 119:1239–1247
19. Tosti A, Piraccini BM, Pazzaglia M, Vincenzi C (2003) Clobetasol propionate 0,05% under occlusion in the treatment of alopecia areata totalis/universalis. J Am Acad Dermatol 49:96–98
20. Friedland R, Tal R, Lapidoth M, Zuluvnov A, Ben Amitai D (2013) Pulse corticosteroid therapy for alopecia areata in children: a retrospective study. Dermatology 227:37–44
21. Sharma VK, Muralighar S (1998) Treatment of widespread alopecia areata in young patients with monthly oral corticosteroid pulse. Pediatr Dermatol 15:313–317
22. Kim SM, Lee HS, Hann SK (1999) The efficacy of low-dose oral corticosteroids in the treatment of vitiligo patients. Int J Dermatol 38:540–550
23. Pasricha JS, Khaitan BK (1993) Oral mini-pulse therapy with bethametasone in vitiligo patients having extensive or fast-spreading disease. Int J Dermatol 32:753–757
24. Kanwar AJ, Mahajan R, Parsad D (2013) Low-dose oral mini-pulse dexamethasone therapy in progressive unstable vitiligo. J Cutan Med Surg 17:259–268
25. Marqueling AL, Cordoro KM (2013) Systemic treatment for severe pediatric psoriasis. A practical approach. Dermatol Clin 31:267–288
26. Nicolaidou E, Katsambas AD (2003) Antihistamines and steroids in pediatric dermatology. Clin Dermatol 21:321–324
27. Hengge UR, Ruzika T, Schwartz RA, Cork MJ (2006) Adverse effects of topical glucocorticosteroids. J Am Acad Dermatol 54:1–15
28. Feldman RJ, Maibach HI (1967) Regional variation in pecutaneous penetration of 14C cortisol in man. J Invest Dermatol 48:181–183
29. Schmitt J, von Kobyletzki L, Svensson A, Apfelbacher C (2011) Efficacy and tollerability of proactive treatment with topical corticosteroids and calcineurin inhibitors for atopic eczema:

systematic review and meta-analysis of randomized controlled trials. Br J Dermatol 164:415–428

30. Devillers AC, Oranje AP (2006) Efficacy and safety of 'wet-wrap' dressings as an intervention treatment in children with severe and/or refractory atopic dermatitis: a critical review of the literature. Br J Dermatol 154:579–585
31. English JS (2000) Corticosteroid-induced contact dermatitis: a pragmatic approach. Clin Exp Dermatol 25:261–264
32. Aubert-Wastiaux H, Moret L, Le Rhun A, Fontenoy AM, Nguyen JM, Leux C, Misery L, Young P, Chastaing M, Danou N, Lombrail P, Boralevi F, Lacour JP, Mazereeuw-Hautier J, Stalder JF, Barbarot S (2011) Topical corticosteroid phobia in atopic dermatitis: a study of its nature, origins and frequency. Br J Dermatol 165:808–814

Corticosteroids in Pediatric Endocrinology

Cosimo Giannini and Angelika Mohn

Introduction

Glucocorticoids, the end products of the hypothalamic–pituitary–adrenal axis, are human steroid hormones secreted by the zona fasciculata of the adrenal cortex (Fig. 1). This class of steroids is essential for the physiological and daily maintenance and regulation of the balance between basal and stress-related homeostasis [22, 52]. Several biologic processes in virtually all physiological organ systems are mediated and influenced by this class of molecules [22, 52]. Glucocorticoids are also essential for the proper functioning of almost all organs and tissues of the organism, including the central nervous and cardiovascular systems and metabolic organs, such as the liver and adipose tissue, as well as the immune/inflammatory response [22, 52]. In addition, glucocorticoids at "pharmacologic" or "stress-related" doses are irreplaceable therapeutic means for many allergic, inflammatory, autoimmune, and lymphoproliferative diseases [90]. Moreover, glucocorticoids are used for the treatment of a wide spectrum of disorders in childhood. In particular, glucocorticoid replacement remains the cornerstone of treatment for life-threatening endocrinopathies in childhood, such as congenital adrenal hyperplasia, Addison disease, and steroid replacement therapy for subjects with secondary hypothalamic–pituitary–adrenal axis deficit. The normal physiology of cortisol secretion and metabolism has been the focus of much research, the results and limitations of which are relevant to the consideration of optimal glucocorticoid replacement therapy in childhood. They challenge assumptions about the dose and pattern of glucocorticoid replacement, the choice of which glucocorticoid to use, and the use of reference ranges or targets in assessing glucocorticoid replacement therapy in patients with hypocortisolemia. Therefore, in-depth knowledge of the physiological

C. Giannini, MD, PhD • A. Mohn, MD (✉)
Department of Pediatrics, University of Chieti, Via dei Vestini 5, I, Chieti 66100, Italy
e-mail: amohn@unich.it

R. Cimaz (ed.), *Systemic Corticosteroids for Inflammatory Disorders in Pediatrics*, DOI 10.1007/978-3-319-16056-6_11

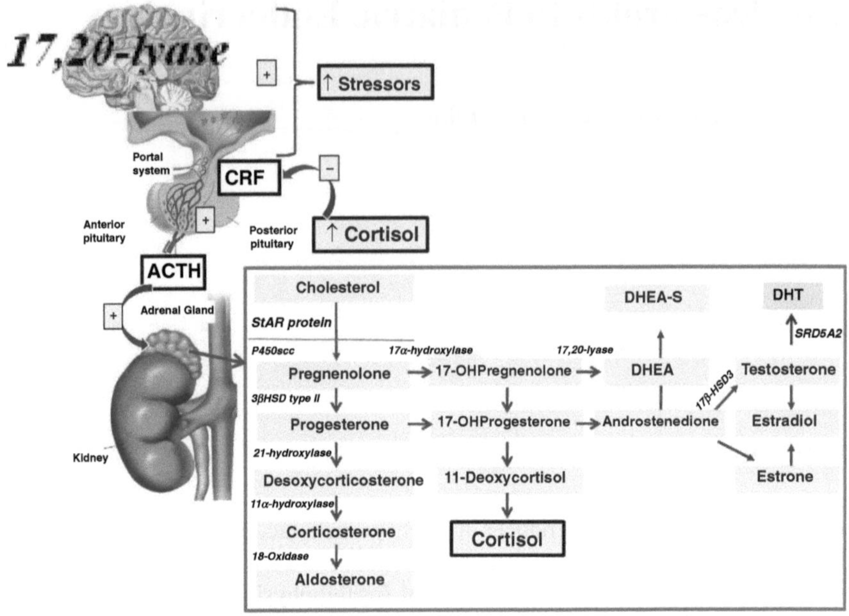

Fig. 1 Regulation of the hypothalamic–pituitary–adrenal axis. Adrenal cortisol production and secretion are regulated by the hypothalamic–pituitary–adrenal axis. Basal diurnal rhythm (regulated by internal clock genes) and various stress factors prompt the release of corticotropin-releasing hormone (*CRH*), which stimulates production and secretion of adrenocorticotropin (*ACTH*) from the pituitary gland. ACTH then stimulates cortisol (and androgen) production and release from the zona fasciculata and the zona reticularis. Positive feed-forward regulation pathways are highlighted. Negative feedback control to the hypothalamus and the pituitary gland works directly through cortisol

pattern of cortisol production and action as well as of the therapeutic opportunity can be challenging for physicians, pediatricians, and pediatric endocrinologists. In this chapter the physiology of the hypothalamic–pituitary–adrenal axis and of glucocorticoids is described. In addition, glucocorticoid replacement therapy in the main clinical disorders in youths (i.e., congenital adrenal hyperplasia, Addison disease, and Cushing disease) is elucidated.

Adrenal Gland: Embryology and Physiology

The adrenal gland was first described in 1552 by Bartolomeu Estaquio as the "glandulae renis incumbents" in *Opuscula Anatômica* [42], although its function remained a mystery for centuries. The mystery began to be solved in 1885, however, when Thomas Addison described the clinical features of 11 patients with primary adrenal insufficiency [57]. In 1949, the synthesis of cortisone facilitated the treatment of this condition [50]. The adrenal gland is made of two tissue types, namely, the adrenal medulla and the adrenal cortex, which have different embryonic origins. By 4–5 weeks of gestation, cells from the mesoderm aggregate to form a primitive cortex between the posterior part of the dorsal mesentery and the gonadal ridge [7]. Shortly thereafter, this primitive cortex becomes surrounded by a narrow band of cells termed the permanent cortex. By 7–8 weeks of fetal life, the primitive cortex is invaded by chromaffin cells that develop rapidly and eventually replace most of the primitive cortex, forming the medulla. At this time the adrenal gland is close to the cranial part of the primitive kidney and not far from the genital ridge. The adrenal medulla, which originates from ectodermal cells, has an entirely different function from the mesodermal adrenal cortex.

In mammals, the adrenal cortex is made of three zones. The first region is the outer zone, the zona glomerulosa, which is responsible for the production and secretion of the mineralocorticoid aldosterone. The inner region is divided into the zona fasciculata and the zona reticularis and is responsible for synthesis and production of glucocorticoids (cortisol, corticosterone, and adrenal androgens). We first focus our discussion on the physiological function and regulation of cortisol production. Then we consider the more common disorders related to primary or secondary hypocortisolism, their potential therapeutic approach, and therapy-related complications in childhood.

Biosynthesis of Cortisol

Cortisol is the principal glucocorticoid hormone produced by the adrenal cortex in humans. The production of cortisol is the result of a series of reactions that involve the concerted action of several enzymes within the adrenals. In this complex process of steroidogenesis, the uptake of cholesterol to the mitochondria represents the first and critical step that is facilitated by the action of a regulatory protein called the steroidogenic acute regulatory protein [75]. The biosynthetic pathway of the adrenal steroids is shown in Fig. 1. Thus, during steroidogenesis, cholesterol is the precursor of a number of steroid hormones of both gonadal and adrenocortical origin. Although they share similar chemical formulae, small differences in their molecular structure characterize each steroid hormone and give them specific functions [86]. The pathway from cholesterol to the end steroid products requires five cytochrome P450 enzymes [cholesterol side-chain cleavage enzyme (20-hydroxylase, 22-hydroxylase, 20,22-lyase, CYP11A), 3β-hydroxysteroid dehydrogenase (3β-HSD), 17α-hydroxylase and 17,20-lyase (CYP17), 21-hydroxylase (CYP21), 11β-hydroxylase (CYP11B1), aldosterone synthetase (11β-hydroxylation, 18-hydroxylation, 18-oxidation, CYP11B)]. Cholesterol is stored in the adrenal cell as cholesterol esters [75, 86]. Under the influence of an esterase, cholesterol becomes available and is transported to the mitochondria, where it is converted into pregnenolone [75, 86]. This steroid then moves into the endoplasmic reticulum, where 3β-hydroxysteroid dehydrogenase, 21-hydroxylase, and 17-3β-hydroxylase enzymes are located. The resulting steroids include 11-deoxycorticosterone (DOC) and 11-deoxycortisol as well as two C-19 carbon steroids, androstenedione and dehydroepiandrosterone. At this point, DOC and 11-deoxycortisol return to the mitochondria, where they are converted into corticosterone and cortisol, respectively. This is the end of the biosynthetic process in the cells of the fasciculata. In the cells of the zona glomerulosa in the mitochondria, DOC is transformed into corticosterone, 18-hydroxycorticosterone, and aldosterone [75, 86].

Control of Corticosteroid Secretion

Synthesis and secretion of cortisol are regulated by the pituitary hormone adrenocorticotropin (ACTH), which in turn is regulated by hypothalamic corticotropin-releasing hormone (CRH) with the synergistic action of arginine vasopressin (AVP). These hormones comprise the hypothalamic–pituitary–adrenal axis that is directly related to a complex closed-loop system. Indeed, CRH is synthesized in the hypothalamus and carried to the anterior pituitary, where it stimulates ACTH release. Finally, ACTH stimulates the adrenal cortex to secrete cortisol. Cortisol inhibits the synthesis and secretion of both CRH and ACTH in a negative feedback regulation system [64, 67, 85, 109].

CRH is a 41-amino acid straight-chain peptide secreted mainly by the median eminence into the portal vessels. Via specific receptors (CRH-R1), CRH activates the formation of cyclic adenosine monophosphate, which then activates a series of protein kinases, resulting in increased transcription of the pro-opiomelanocortin gene and in ACTH formation [12, 64, 67, 85, 109]. ACTH has a half-life in blood of a few minutes and like other hormones binds specific receptors on the adrenal cortex, type 2 melanocortin receptors (MC2-R), and increases cyclic adenosine monophosphate formation to initiate the synthesis of cortisol, which is released immediately into the systemic circulation by diffusion [12, 64, 67, 85, 109]. ACTH stimulation of cortisol on the adrenal includes both an immediate and a chronic phase. Acutely, over a few minutes, steroidogenesis is stimulated through a steroidogenic acute regulatory protein (STAR-)-mediated increase in cholesterol delivery to the CYP11A1 enzyme in the inner mitochondrial membrane [14]. In the more chronic phase, over 24–26 h of exposure, ACTH leads to an increase in the synthesis of all steroidogenic CYP enzymes (CYP11A1, CYP17, CYP21A2, CYP11B1) in addition to adrenodoxin, and these effects are mediated at the transcriptional level. Additional effects of ACTH include: (a) increased synthesis of the low-density lipoprotein and high-density lipoprotein receptors, and possibly also HMG-CoA (3-hydroxy-3-methyl-glutaryl-CoA) reductase, the rate-limiting step in cholesterol biosynthesis; (b) increased adrenal weight by inducing both hyperplasia and hypertrophy [12, 14, 64, 67, 85, 109].

Glucocorticoid synthesis is mostly affected by two variables: the secretion patterns and the secretion rate. The former is related to three main physiological mechanisms affecting the secretion of cortisol: pulsative secretion and diurnal variation, stress, and negative feedback. The normal pattern of glucocorticoid secretion includes both a diurnal rhythm and a pulsatile ultradian rhythm. In fact, the natural cortisol peak in humans occurs early, before awakening, and falls progressively during the day, reaching low levels in the evening [9, 112]. The circadian rhythm of glucocorticoid secretion is accompanied by a pulsatile ultradian rhythm throughout the 24-h cycle [20]. As documented by automated frequent blood-sampling techniques, the pulses vary in amplitude throughout the day, with the amplitude generally decreasing during the diurnal trough. Of note, the two components are separable secretory modes. Thus the "pulsatile" and "circadian" rhythms are independently regulated [118]. Ultradian rhythmicity has been shown in rats [116], monkeys [94], and humans [9, 38, 46, 112]. Among the most relevant practical consequences [118] of the pulsatility is that the underlying pattern of spontaneous pulses might not be detected if sampling is infrequent and/or conducted over a short period. This might also have an additional effect on the tissue specificity. In fact, the two glucocorticoid-related tissue receptors have different affinities. Therefore, according to the circulating level of ligands, the receptors will be differentially occupied and activated [118], especially affecting the occupancy of the lower-affinity glucocorticoids receptors [118]. Prolonged versus intermittent exposure seems to also affect steroid-responsive hepatic enzymes. Studies have documented that short exposure to glucocorticoids may have different effects on tyrosine aminotransferase, an enzyme involved in the catalysis of the first step in tyrosine catabolism [88, 107]. Finally, prolonged exposure to glucocorticoids has been shown to downregulate glucocorticoids receptors [88].

This complex regulation system is further characterized by the ability of the adrenal glands to secrete steroids in a stress-related way [37]. Surgical stress such as trauma and tissue destruction, medical stress such as acute illness, fever, and hypoglycemia, and emotional stress related to psychological upset result in a significant increase in cortisol secretion in most cases. The hypothalamic–pituitary–adrenal axis in conjunction with the sympathetic system connects the brain with the periphery of the body. Of note, the body responses to a stressor – physical or emotional – that disrupts the homeostatic balance of the organism are mainly related to the hypothalamic–pituitary–adrenal axis activity [37, 93]. All the complex activities characterizing the individual's adaptive response to excessive stress are stereotypical and usually defined as the "general adaptation syndrome" [37, 93]. This physiological response involves interactions between hormones and the central nervous system. Glucocorticoids along with catecholamines (the end product of sympathetic nervous system activation) secreted by the adrenal medulla and sympathetic nerves orchestrate the "fight or flight" response, which is the first stage of the general adaptation syndrome [69]. The fight or flight response refers to different factors including: a quick mobilization of energy from storage to different systems, such as the heart, muscles, and the brain; a prompt transport of nutrients and oxygen to relevant tissues facilitated by accelerated cardiac output and breathing rate; and increased blood pressure [23]. According to the theory of Munck and colleagues [77], the physiological function of stress-induced increase in glucocorticoid levels is to defend the body against the normal defense reactions that are activated by stress and not against the stress itself. According to this theory, glucocorticoids accomplish this function by turning off these defense reactions, thus preventing them from overshooting and threatening homeostasis. Therefore, it is now commonly accepted that glucocorticoid secretion in a stress situation plays a double and complementary function: a permissive and suppressive effect, the former preparing or priming defense mechanisms for action and the latter limiting these actions [78]. CRH and AVP neurons of the hypothalamic paraventricular nuclei and the noradrenergic neurons of the locus coeruleus/norepinephrine–central sympathetic systems in the brain stem represent the main apparatus of the stress system. In addition, the peripheral branches of this system consist of the hypothalamic–pituitary–adrenal axis and the systemic sympathetic and adrenomedullary nervous system [21]. Both central components of the stress system are stimulated by cholinergic and serotonergic neurotransmitters and inhibited by γ-aminobutyric acid, benzodiazepine, and arcuate nucleus pro-opiomelanocortin peptides [19, 31]. Activation of the central stress system results in the secretion of CRH and AVP into the hypophyseal portal circulation, thus inducing glucocorticoid secretion by the hypothalamic–pituitary–adrenal axis. In this complex event the systemic sympathetic and adrenomedullary nervous systems are also activated as a direct consequence of central stress system stimulation, which in turn results in a peripheral secretion of catecholamines and several neuropeptides. At rest the stress system is still active, assisting the body in responding to various distinct signals, for example, circadian, neurosensory, blood-borne, and limbic [22]. The activation of the stress system has thus several effects: it increases arousal, accelerates motor reflexes, improves attention and cognitive function, decreases appetite and sexual arousal, and also increases the tolerance of pain [23]. Although these types of stress are well known to affect cortisol production, research is still ongoing to define all the regulatory mechanisms involved. Among the reported results, studies of the immune system have shown that leukocytes may play a relevant regulatory action by secreting a series of interleukins able to significantly affect the adrenal axis [110].

The negative feedback represents a relevant feedback control able to constantly equilibrate the secretion rate of both ACTH and cortisol. When plasma concentrations of cortisol increase markedly, a negative feedback effect on the secretion of CRH and ACTH is induced [64, 67, 85, 109].

The secretion rate and cortisol metabolism represent an additional variable that needs to be considered in defining glucocorticoid synthesis in the young. The daily cortisol production rate ranges between 5 and 10 mg/m^2 body surface area [16, 28, 51, 55]. Circulating cortisol in humans is about 90 % plasma protein bound, mostly to cortisol-binding globulin and less to albumin, while only 5–10 % circulates unbound as a free active hormone [64, 67, 85, 109]. The free cortisol concentration ranges from approximately 1 nmol/l at the diurnal trough to approximately 100 nmol/l at the diurnal peak [96]. Estimations of the circulating half-life of cortisol vary between 70 and 120 min. Cortisol is cleared through several distinct pathways, including A-ring reduction to form tetrahydrocortisol and its 5α-isomer, allotetrahydrocortisol, hydroxylation to yield 6-β-hydroxycortisol, and the reduction of the 20-oxo group to produce cortisol [34]. Cortisone is an inactive steroid that circulates at concentrations of around 60 nmol/l, largely unbound to plasma proteins and without marked diurnal variation. The main source of cortisone is 11-β-hydroxysteroid dehydrogenase-type 2 (11-β-HSD-2) in the kidney [96, 108], which gates glucocorticoid access to nuclear receptors by a prereceptor mechanism. 11-β-HSD-1 converts cortisone to cortisol, amplifying the steroid signal in target cells [97]. Additionally, cortisol derives from circulating cortisone via conversion in peripheral tissues expressing the enzyme 11-β-HSD-1. The cortisol secretion rate in children also shows some peculiarities. Several studies in children have shown that in normal children and adolescents, the cortisol secretion rate is directly related to body size [28, 51, 74]. Migeon et al. showed that when the values are corrected for body surface area, the rates are similar at various ages; in fact, the average ± standard deviation was 12 ± 2 with a range of 8–16 mg/m^2/24 h [74]. Using stable isotope dilution/mass spectroscopy, Esteban et al. showed that the cortisol secretion rate for 12 normal subjects was lower, accounting for 5.7 ± 1.5 mg/m^2/24 h [74]. Kerrigan et al. also investigated the daily cortisol production and clearance rates in a group of 18 normal unstressed pubertal male subjects by applying deconvolution analysis to serum cortisol concentrations obtained every 20 min for 24 h [51] and found similar results to Esteban's data. In addition, they showed that the estimated cortisol production rate for the early puberty group was indistinguishable from that of the late puberty subjects [51]. No difference was observed between the two pubertal groups in the secretory burst frequency and half-duration, mass of cortisol released per secretory episode, average maximal rate of hormone secretion, and serum cortisol half-life [51]. A significant diurnal pattern of cortisol secretion was observed for all subjects, manifested by nyctohemeral variations in the frequency of adrenocortical secretory bursts, the amplitude (maximal rate of cortisol secretion) and the mass of cortisol released per secretory episode. In this age group, maximum serum hormone concentrations occurred between 07:06 and 11:14 h [51]. Similar results were also reported by Linder et al., who evaluated the cortisol production rate in 33 normal children and adolescents, using a stable isotope-dilution technique with high-performance liquid chromatography-mass spectrometry [61].

Effects of Cortisol

Glucocorticoids are essential for the maintenance of homeostasis and enable the organism to prepare for, respond to, and manage physical or emotional stress. These hormones affect nearly every organ and tissue in the body and have diverse life-sustaining effects throughout the life span. Glucocorticoid access to nuclear receptors is gated by the 11-β-HSD enzymes. Corticosteroids are highly lipophilic and are thought to diffuse readily across biological membranes to access their intracellular receptors [41, 81]. At the cellular level, the myriad effects of corticosteroids are largely a consequence of transcriptional actions mediated via binding to two types of intracellular receptors: the high-affinity mineralocorticoid receptor and the lower-affinity glucocorticoid receptors [32, 70]. On binding ligand, glucocorticoid receptors and mineralocorticoid receptors dissociate from complexes with chaperone proteins, translocate to the nucleus, and bind directly or indirectly to the regulatory regions of target genes: ≈2 % of the human genome is regulated by glucocorticoids [89], although few, any genes are exclusively controlled by corticosteroids. Rapid glucocorticoid signaling via membrane binding has also been postulated [18].

Cortisol is involved in peripheral glucose uptake and utilization (gluconeogenesis and glycogenolysis). Cortisol also affects the maintenance of proper cardiovascular tone, endothelial integrity, and the distribution of fluids within the vascular compartment. Moreover, cortisol potentiates the vasoconstrictor action of catecholamines and decreases the production of nitric oxide [25, 36]. Therefore, cortisol deficiency results in hypoglycemia, hypotension, lethargy, decreased appetite, absolute leukocytosis, eosinophilia, and anemia. Cortisol influences the activity and direction of the reactions underlying intermediary metabolism and many functions of the central nervous system, including arousal, cognition, mood, and sleep. Physiological amounts of glucocorticoids are also essential for normal renal tubular function and thus for water and electrolyte homeostasis. Studies have shown that 15–20 % of the human leukocyte transcriptome is influenced by glucocorticoids [24, 33], and almost two thirds of them are induced, whereas the rest are suppressed. Through their genomic actions, glucocorticoids regulate cellular metabolism primarily through catabolic actions in the liver, muscle, and adipose tissue [24, 33]. Finally, multiple components regulating the quantity and quality of immune/inflammatory responses are well-recognized glucocorticoid targets, providing the basis for the wide use of glucocorticoids as potent anti-inflammatory/immunosuppressive drugs in the treatment of inflammatory diseases and cancer [90].

Cortisol Replacement Therapy: Relevance in Pediatric Endocrinology

The first treatment for adrenal insufficiency was introduced in the 1930s when lipid extracts from adrenal glands were tested, leading to a drastic and rapid drop of the mortality rate from 100 % to a seemingly normal life expectancy. In 1937 and 1949, the synthesis of 11-deoxycortisone (11-DOC) and cortisone, respectively, represented major improvements in therapy. Since the first published report of the efficacy of cortisone in the treatment of rheumatoid arthritis in 1949 [92], patients with adrenal insufficiency have been treated with glucocorticoid replacement, and after the introduction of fludrocortisone in the 1950s replacement therapy has remained virtually unchanged [66]. Hydrocortisone is now used in many centers around the world.

As mentioned, following the first report of the efficacy of cortisone in treating rheumatoid arthritis, glucocorticoids have been used widely in several autoimmune diseases and in the treatment of a spectrum of disorders in childhood. In particular, glucocorticoid replacement remains the cornerstone of treatment for certain life-threatening endocrinopathies in childhood, such as congenital adrenal hyperplasia, Addison disease, and as replacement therapy for those subjects with secondary hypothalamic–pituitary–adrenal axis deficit. In the next sections, a short description of these main disorders in childhood is provided, evidencing the role of glucocorticoids in their treatment.

Adrenal Insufficiency

Adrenal insufficiency is a clinical condition characterized by a state of failure of the adrenal cortex to provide sufficient amounts of steroid hormones, in particular glucocorticoids. Several causes might be responsible for the development of adrenal insufficiency in childhood. According to the localization of its underlying cause, adrenal insufficiency in childhood can be essentially categorized into two major groups: primary and secondary. The most frequent causes of primary and secondary adrenal insufficiency are summarized in Table 1.

The group of primary adrenal insufficiency includes: autoimmune adrenalitis (Addison disease, which can arise in isolation or as part of an autoimmune polyglandular syndrome), infections (tuberculosis, cryptococcosis, mycosis, AIDS), congenital conditions (adrenoleukodystrophy, adrenomyeloneuropathy, congenital adrenal hyperplasia), bilateral adrenalectomy, bilateral adrenal hemorrhage, metastases and surgery, and drug-induced adrenal insufficiency (treatment with mitotane, etomidate, ketoconazole, aminoglutethimide). Secondary adrenal insufficiency results from hypothalamic–pituitary impairment, with consecutive lack of CRH and/or ACTH. Thus, this group mainly includes: pituitary tumors or other tumors of the hypothalamic–pituitary region often associated with panhypopituitarism (caused

Table 1 Most frequent causes of primary and secondary adrenal insufficiency

Primary	Autoimmune adrenalitis (isolated or related to an autoimmune polyglandular syndrome)
	Infections (tuberculosis, cryptococcosis, mycosis, AIDS)
	Congenital (congenital adrenal hyperplasia, adrenoleukodystrophy, adrenomyeloneuropathy)
	Bilateral adrenalectomy
	Bilateral adrenal hemorrhage
	Metastases and surgery
	Drug-induced adrenal insufficiency (treatment with mitotane, etomidate, ketoconazole, aminoglutethimide)
Secondary	Pituitary tumors or other tumors of the hypothalamic–pituitary axis (secondary adrenal insufficiency as a consequences of tumor growth and treatment, i.e., surgery, radiation
	Exogenous chronic glucocorticoid treatment
	Head trauma
	Pituitary infiltration (tuberculosis, sarcoidosis, Wegener's granulomatosis)

by tumor growth or treatment with surgery or irradiation), exogenous glucocorticoids leading to suppression of CRH/ACTH release, head trauma, and pituitary infiltration.

Although most of these conditions rarely occur in childhood, adrenal insufficiency related to congenital adrenal hyperplasia, Addison disease, and Cushing's syndrome are not uncommon, thus requiring clinicians, health-care planners, and patients to understand these life-threatening disorders and the proper management of adrenal insufficiency in the various clinical settings. While etiological aspects characterize the different causes of adrenal insufficiency, glucocorticoids traditionally represent the main therapeutic option in all forms of adrenal insufficiency, including acute and chronic states.

Acute adrenal insufficiency is a life-threatening disease that involves severe hypotension or hypovolemia, acute abdominal pain, nausea and vomiting, lack of stamina, and weight loss [4]. Anorexia, fever, weakness, fatigue, lethargy, and confusion may also be associated with this condition. Dizziness, irritability, and postural hypotension are frequent complaints; these symptoms can be triggered by several predisposing factors such as trauma, surgery, and infections, which suddenly increase the need for corticosteroids. Acute adrenal insufficiency-related shock is often unresponsive to volume replacement and vasoconstrictor agents [54, 84, 111]. Hyperpigmentation and salt-craving are also often detected. According to the underlying cause, the onset of the disease can be insidious, taking years to diagnose, or can lead to the development of an acute crisis following an intercurrent illness [54, 84].

Congenital Adrenal Hyperplasia

Congenital adrenal hyperplasia (CAH) is an autosomal recessive disorder caused by the deficiency of an enzyme involved in steroidogenesis within the adrenal cortex [72, 115]. Although several enzymatic defects have been described, the most common is cytochrome P450 21-hydroxylase (CYP21) deficiency. The defect accounts for approximately 95 % of cases and results from mutations [5, 44, 56, 103] of the *CYP21A2* gene located on chromosome 6p21.3. The enzyme adrenal insufficiency converts 17-hydroxyprogesterone into 11-deoxycortisol and progesterone into 11-deoxycortisone, which are precursors for cortisol and aldosterone, respectively (Fig. 1). Therefore, defects of the enzymatic activity result in an impaired adrenal synthesis of cortisol often associated with aldosterone deficiency, which in turn leads to increased ACTH secretion by the pituitary gland. The impaired cortisol/aldosterone synthesis and the increased ACTH production directly induce: severe salt wasting (SW) and Addisonian crisis, related to cortisol and aldosterone deficiency; adrenal gland hyperplasia, related to ACTH oversecretion; and accumulation of steroid precursors, inducing a variable degree of virilization as a direct consequence of adrenal androgen overproduction [115].

According to the degree of the enzyme deficiency, different clinical phenotypes can be defined including: classic SW, classic simple virilizing (SV), and nonclassic (NC) CAH. The classic SW form is the most severe form of enzymatic activity deficiency, resulting from a residual activity of less than 1 %. In this form, severe cortisol deficiency and decreased aldosterone synthesis are detected. Female patients are virilized prenatally owing to adrenal androgen excess. Neonates (boys and girls) also suffer from life-threatening Addisonian crisis. In those forms characterized by a residual enzyme activity of 1–2 % (simple virilizing) CAH, the residual activity is enough for sufficient aldosterone production, thus preventing SW. By contrast, cortisol synthesis is impaired and this results in the development of genital ambiguity in affected female patients due to prenatal virilization. In those forms with a residual enzymatic activity around 20–50 % (nonclassic), cortisol and aldosterone production are normal. In these subjects a mild androgen excess may be detected and may induce premature pubarche, cystic acne, hirsutism, and menstrual disorders in some subjects in childhood/adolescence, or may even be asymptomatic. Some patients present first in adulthood with fertility problems.

Addison Disease

Autoimmune adrenalitis, or autoimmune Addison disease (AAD), is a rare condition in childhood. Both humoral and cellular immunity play a role in AAD pathogenesis, with presence of adrenal cortex autoantibodies in the serum of patients [3]. These adrenal cortex autoantibodies are of the immunoglobulin subclasses IgG1, IgG2, and IgG4 and are directed against the steroidogenic enzymes, with steroidogenic 21-hydroxylase being the most prevalent [100, 117]. Although the presence of adrenal cortex autoantibodies is a main feature of the disease, their role in the pathogenesis of autoimmune Addison disease is still debated. Studies have shown that the destruction of adrenocortical cells is mainly mediated by T-lymphocytes. Thus the secondary release of peptides may result in the production of antibodies [13]. Autoimmune adrenalitis may present in 60 % of cases as part of an autoimmune polyendocrine syndrome, while in the remaining 40 % it is isolated [4]. During the first two decades of life, isolated AAD is predominantly observed in male subjects (70 %); however, after the third decade of life, there is a substantial female preponderance (81 %) [102]. Spontaneous recovery of adrenal function has been described but is rare. Addison disease is the final result of AAD; the initial phase is subclinical, and after at least 90 % of the adrenal gland has been destroyed, symptoms of adrenal failure occur [11]. This condition can easily be misdiagnosed in childhood, thus negatively affecting data on its true prevalence; autoimmune adrenalitis is the main cause of adrenal insufficiency after the introduction of antituberculosis therapy, and is responsible for 68–94 % of the cases in European and North American reports [10, 29, 79]. Determination of inappropriately low cortisol production associated with the presence of high titers of adrenal cortex autoantibodies is strongly suggestive of autoimmune adrenalitis. The diagnosis is confirmed by excluding other causes of adrenal failure, using other tests as necessary. Treatment is based on corticosteroid replacement, and the prognosis following treatment is the same as for the normal population. Thus the standard initial therapy is corticosteroid replacement.

Cushing's Syndrome in Children: Role of Glucocorticoid Therapy

Cushing's syndrome refers to a large group of clinical conditions characterized by the presence of signs and symptoms associated with prolonged exposure to inappropriate levels of the hormone cortisol [67]. In children with Cushing's syndrome, the hypothalamic–pituitary–adrenal axis has lost its ability for self-regulation. Thus, the impaired hypothalamic–pituitary–adrenal axis function may result from an excessive secretion of either ACTH or cortisol and from the loss of the negative feedback function [67].

Cushing's syndrome is a rare entity; its overall incidence is approximately two to five new cases per million people per year. Characteristically, in older children, a female predominance has been described that decreases with younger age and seems to switch to a male predominance in infants and young toddlers [67, 85, 109].

Although both exogenous and endogenous causes can induce Cushing's syndrome, the former are certainly more common in children. In particular, exogenous or iatrogenic causes might result from chronic administration of glucocorticoids or ACTH (such as in the treatment of many nonendocrine diseases including neoplastic, hematologic, pulmonary, autoimmune, epileptic, and dermatologic disorders). Among the endogenous causes of Cushing's syndrome in children, ACTH overproduction from the pituitary (called Cushing's disease) is the most common, and results from an ACTH-secreting pituitary microadenoma or, rarely, a macroadenoma. Cushing's disease is more common in children older than 7 years of age, accounting for approximately 75 % of all cases of Cushing's syndrome in this age group. By contrast, in children younger than 7 years adrenal causes of Cushing's syndrome (adenoma, carcinoma, or bilateral hyperplasia) are the most frequent. Ectopic ACTH/CRH production occurs rarely in young children and adolescents, and for some forms they have never been described in young children [85, 104, 105, 109]. A few additional rare diseases, such as primary pigmented adrenocortical nodular disease (PPNAD), massive macronodular adrenal hyperplasia (MMAD), McCune–Albright syndrome, might be related to Cushing's syndrome in childhood. PPNAD is a genetic disorder and the majority of cases are associated with Carney complex, a syndrome of multiple endocrine abnormalities in addition to lentigo and myxomas. Periodic, cyclical, or otherwise atypical Cushing's syndrome is often documented in children and adolescents with PPNAD. MMAD is another rare bilateral disease that leads to Cushing's syndrome [105]. In children with MMAD, the adrenal glands are massively enlarged, with multiple huge nodules that are typical yellow-to-brown cortisol-producing adenomas. Data have shown that in some patients with MMAD, cortisol levels seem to increase with food ingestion (food-dependent Cushing's syndrome), which might result from an aberrant expression of the gastric inhibitory polypeptide receptor in the adrenal glands. In the majority of patients with MMAD, however, the disease does not appear to be gastric inhibitory polypeptide receptor dependent.

In children with McCune–Albright syndrome, adrenal adenomas or, more frequently, bilateral macronodular adrenal hyperplasia can also be seen [30, 53]. In this syndrome, there is a somatic mutation of the *GNAS1* gene leading to constitutive activation of the Gsα protein and continuous, non-ACTH-dependent activation of steroidogenesis by the adrenal cortex.

The treatment of choice varies according to the underlying cause [49, 85, 104, 105, 109]. Transsphenoidal surgery (TSS) with or without irradiation of the pituitary gland represents the treatment of choice for almost all patients with ACTH-secreting pituitary adenomas (Cushing's disease). Surgical resection with or without radiotherapy is also the treatment of choice for benign adrenal tumors. The treatment of choice in bilateral micronodular or macronodular adrenal disease, such as PPNAD and MMAD, is usually bilateral total adrenalectomy. In addition, in subjects with Cushing's disease or ectopic ACTH-dependent Cushing's syndrome in whom surgery or radiotherapy has failed, or in whom the tumor has not been localized, adrenalectomy is a potential treatment. Finally, pharmacotherapy is also an option if surgery fails for Cushing's disease or in ectopic ACTH secretion where the source cannot be identified. Several molecules can be used, such as mitotane, aminoglutethimide, metyrapone, trilostane, and ketoconazole, which may act by: inhibiting the biosynthesis of corticosteroids by blocking the action of 11-β-hydroxylase and cholesterol side chain cleavage enzymes; destroying adrenocortical cells that secrete cortisol; blocking the conversion of cholesterol to pregnenolone in the adrenal cortex; inhibiting the synthesis of cortisol, aldosterone, and androgens; preventing the conversion of 11-deoxycortisol to cortisol; inhibiting the conversion of pregnenolone to progesterone; or blocking adrenal steroidogenesis.

Although the treatment of choice varies according to the underlying cause of Cushing's syndrome or disease, the hypothalamic–pituitary–adrenal axis is often negatively affected [49, 85, 104, 105, 109]. Hypopituitarism is the most common adverse effect, and it is more frequent when surgery precedes radiotherapy. In addition, after the completion of successful TSS in Cushing's disease or excision of an autonomously functioning adrenal adenoma, there will be a period of adrenal insufficiency while the hypothalamic–pituitary–adrenal axis recovers. Therefore, in this situation glucocorticoids might be replaced. Treatment is aimed at restoring physiological changes, with a usual replacement dose of 12–15 mg/m^2/day two or three times daily [63]. In addition, in the immediate postoperative period, cortisol treatment should be started initially at stress doses of glucocorticoids and then weaning relatively rapidly to a physiological replacement dose.

According to the underlying alteration, glucocorticoid replacement might be temporarily adopted only for a short period [49, 85, 104, 105, 109]. Thereafter, patients should be closely followed up with a systematic assessment of the adrenocortical function. Clinicians might consider discontinuing glucocorticoid treatment if normal responses to a 1-h ACTH test are documented (cortisol level over 18 μg/dl at 30 or 60 min after ACTH stimulation) [49, 85, 104, 105, 109].

In children with unilateral adrenalectomy as in patients with Cushing's disease post-TSS, a similar replacement regimen is needed for a single adrenocortical tumor. By contrast, for those who have undergone bilateral adrenalectomy, lifetime replacement with both glucocorticoids (as described previously) and mineralocorticoids (fludrocortisone 0.1–0.3 mg daily) is needed. In these patients, too, glucocorticoids at stress doses are needed immediately postoperatively, with a relatively quick weaning to physiological replacement doses. In addition, for temporary and permanent adrenal insufficiency, acute illness, trauma, or surgical procedures, stress doses must be adopted in all patients [49, 85, 104, 105, 109].

Replacement Therapy in Young Patients with Impaired Adrenal Function

The main aim of treatment of adrenal insufficiency in childhood is to restore the impaired hypothalamic–pituitary–adrenal axis, without impairing growth while allowing for normal pubertal development and fertility. In addition, in subjects with congenital adrenal hyperplasia a proper suppression of androgen production is needed to minimize the peripheral effects of hyperandrogenism secretion.

The available evidence suggests that conventional treatment of patients with hypoadrenalism may result in adverse effects on some surrogate markers of disease risk, such as a lower bone mineral density, than in age- and sex-matched controls, and in increased postprandial glucose and insulin concentrations. Although the quality of life of patients with hypoadrenalism may be impaired, there is no evidence of an improvement with higher doses of steroids, although quality of life is better if the hydrocortisone dose is split up, with the highest dose taken in the morning. Thus the evidence suggests that most patients may safely be treated with a low dose of glucocorticoids in two or three divided doses, along with education about the appropriate course of action in the event of intercurrent illnesses.

The glucocorticoid of choice in childhood is hydrocortisone, which is short acting and hence has the lowest growth-suppressing effect (Table 2) [48, 101]. During infancy, especially in subjects needing an initial reduction of markedly elevated adrenal sex hormones, up to 25 mg of hydrocortisone/m^2 may be required. This is more than the daily physiological secretion of 7–9 mg/m^2 in newborns and 6–8 mg/

Table 2 Suggested maintenance therapy for growing patients

Medication	Total dose	Daily doses
Hydrocortisone	15–25 (mg/m^2/day)	Three times per day
Fludrocortisone	0.05–0.2 (mg/m^2/day)	One to two times per day
Sodium chloride supplements	1–3 g/day (1,751 mEq/day)	Divided in several feeding

m^2 in older infants and children [48, 101]. Hydrocortisone oral suspension is not recommended [73]; divided or crushed tablets of hydrocortisone should be used in growing children. Cortisone acetate requires conversion to cortisol for bioactivity [82]; thus hydrocortisone is considered the drug of first choice. To mimic the circadian cortisol secretion, the daily hydrocortisone dose is divided into two or three doses, with administration of one half to two thirds of the total daily dose in the morning. The short elimination half-life of hydrocortisone (approximately 1.5 h) when given in traditional immediate-release preparations, however, leads to high peaks with low values in between. A twice-daily regimen with administration of the second dose 6–8 h after the morning dose is recommended. The timing of the second dose may be changed slightly according to the patient's activities. Some authors postulate that a thrice-daily administration is more beneficial [2, 6, 43, 59, 87], although there is no hard evidence available yet to support this. Whereas hydrocortisone is preferred during infancy and childhood, longer-acting glucocorticoids may be recommended at or near the completion of linear growth, such as in older adolescents or young adults (Table 3). Prednisone and prednisolone should be given twice daily [48, 101]. Prednisolone may be preferable since it is the active drug. The dose (2–4 mg/m^2/day) should be one-fifth that of hydrocortisone. The dosage of dexamethasone is 0.25–0.5 mg/m^2/day given once daily. These steroids have minimal mineralocorticoid effects compared with hydrocortisone. In children with advanced bone age, such as in boys with non-salt-losing CAH, initiation of therapy may precipitate central precocious puberty, requiring additional treatments, such as with a GnRH agonist. In some children with treatment refractory to hydrocortisone, long-acting glucocorticoids may be effective [91]. In symptomatic patients with non-classic-CAH, treatment with glucocorticoids is recommended. In these patients, chronic steroid treatment may suppress the hypothalamic–pituitary–adrenal axis, so they require stress dosing during surgery or severe illness. For asymptomatic patients with non-classic-CAH, hydrocortisone treatment is not required during stress [101]. All patients with classic CAH require mineralocorticoid replacement with fludrocortisone at a dose of 0.05–0.2 mg/day. The dose is slightly higher (up to 0.3 mg/day) in newborns and small infants because of their increased metabolism and end-organ resistance to mineralocorticoids. Such therapy will reduce vasopressin and ACTH levels and lower the dosage of glucocorticoid required. The need for continuing mineralocorticoids should be assessed based on plasma renin activity (PRA) and blood pressure [47]. Although aldosterone levels are normal in patients with NSW CAH, these patients also benefit from mineralocorticoid replacement as

Table 3 Suggested maintenance therapy for fully grown patients

Type of long-acting glucocorticoids	Suggested dose (mg/day)	Daily doses (mg/day)
Hydrocortisone	15–25	Two to three times per day
Prednisone	5–7.5	Two times per day
Prednisolone	0.25–0.5	Two times per day
Dexamethasone	5–50	Once daily
Fludrocortisone	0.05–0.2	Once daily

it helps to decrease the dose of glucocorticoid required to suppress androgens. Hence, published guidelines recommend that all children with classic CAH be treated with fludrocortisone [48, 101]. Owing to the obligatory urinary sodium loss, sodium chloride supplementation should be provided to infants. Sodium chloride supplements are often needed in infancy at 1–3 g/day (17–51 mEq/day; 1 g = 17 mEq of sodium), divided with each feed [48, 76, 101]. Older infants and children generally do not require salt supplementation.

Glucocorticoid Adjustment Issues

Maintenance dosing of glucocorticoids for replacement therapy is based on the need to reproduce the secretory rate of cortisol in the intact system. During severe illness and stress, the activity of the hypothalamic–pituitary–adrenal axis is significantly enhanced, resulting in a considerable rise of cortisol release from the adrenal cortex [4, 36]. Therefore, owing to the relevant changes of glucocorticoid synthesis in different clinical settings, glucocorticoid replacement doses need to be constantly adjusted accordingly. In 2008, a consensus statement for recommendations for the diagnosis and management of corticosteroid insufficiency in critically ill adult patients was published [45, 68]. By contrast, agreement among intensive care and endocrinology specialists is low for the pediatric population, especially regarding diagnostic criteria and the prevalence of adrenal insufficiency associated with critical illness [71, 99]. Pediatric endocrinologists are often required to provide consultation regarding suspected adrenal insufficiency in critically ill children. Although acute adrenal insufficiency is rare, it is a life-threatening condition. Thus early diagnosis is key for effective and life-saving treatment of affected patients. All patients and their partners or relatives must receive crisis prevention training, including a steroid emergency card/bracelet and detailed instructions on stress-related dose adjustment to ensure that medical providers know about their underlying disorder. In addition, an emergency kit must be provided (e.g., 100 mg hydrocortisone-21-hydrogensuccinate) for traveling abroad; alternatively, prednisolone or other corticosteroid preparations can be used in emergency conditions if hydrocortisone is not readily available (Table 4).

Table 4 Recommendations for patients with chronic adrenal failure

Emergency card/bracelet
Education of patient and partner:
Rationale for dose adjustments in stress
Discussion of typical situations requiring dose adjustment (e.g., fever, surgery, trauma)
Nausea, vomiting, and diarrhea as reasons to use parenteral hydrocortisone
Signs and symptoms of emerging adrenal crisis
Provision of a hydrocortisone ampule (e.g., 100 mg hydrocortisone 21-hydrogensuccinate) to the patient for emergency use by attending physician

The cortisol secretory rate increases substantially during physiological stress. Consequently, the complex events that can occur in the setting of an adrenal crisis, mainly characterized by hypoglycemia, hypotension, and even cardiovascular collapse, need to be prevented in patients with adrenal insufficiency (primary or secondary) by adequately educating patients and parents to increase glucocorticoid doses during stress. Although this approach is universally adopted, there is controversy as to what constitutes "stress" and the need to increase glucocorticoid doses. However, the correct definition of a "stressing condition" is of paramount importance for a properly balanced glucocorticoid therapy, thus avoiding preventable episodes of adrenal insufficiency crisis or over-dosages and their associated side effects. If the children act and appear well, they might not require a stress-dose steroid regimen during mild stresses such as immunizations, uncomplicated viral illnesses, and upper respiratory tract infections with sore throat, rhinorrhea, and/or low-grade fever and otitis media. By contrast, clinical conditions such as those accompanied by fever (≥38 °C), vomiting, diarrhea, lethargy, inadequate oral intake, trauma, dental procedures, surgery, and large burns must be considered as "severe stresses," thus requiring an appropriate increase of glucocorticoid doses. In addition, physical exercise and especially moderate to extreme schedules of exercise are also considered "stress" and thus may require glucocorticoid dose increases.

A common recommendation is to treat most stresses that require increased doses with hydrocortisone 30–50 mg/m^2/day (approximately doubling or tripling the daily dose) divided into three or four daily doses [26, 48, 58, 60, 99], with higher doses to cover more severe illnesses or surgical procedures.

Parenteral glucocorticoid administration is indicated for those children who are unable to tolerate oral maintenance or stress doses during an illness. Parents need to be instructed to start at home using 50 mg/m^2 of intramuscular hydrocortisone sodium succinate, which seems to provide coverage for ≈6–8 h. If glucocorticoids are administered intramuscularly, a consultation with a health-care provider is recommended and emergency evaluation and treatment with intravenous hydrocortisone should be undertaken if the child's condition does not improve or if it worsens.

Although it is accepted that patients with hypoadrenalism may also adjust glucocorticoid replacement therapy during moderate to extreme physical activity, the amount of increase is still under debate. The degree to which doses should be increased is also debated, with recommendations varying between two and ten times the maintenance rate [60]. Although some authors postulate that moderate to extreme physical exercise may be facilitated by a slight increase (≈30 %) in hydrocortisone dosage 60 min before exercise [4], there is no evidence to support this. In addition, in a randomized, double-blind crossover study of nine adolescents with congenital adrenal hyperplasia, Weise et al. showed that an additional morning dose of hydrocortisone, which resulted in doubling of cortisol levels, just before short-term high-intensity exercise did not have an effect on blood levels of glucose, lactate, or free fatty acids, on exercise capacity, or on peak blood pressure response [114]. The peak heart rate was marginally (but statistically significantly) higher following the extra dose of hydrocortisone (mean 193 vs. 191 beats/min). Of the nine patients, one correctly identified the session at which he had received the extra dose of hydrocortisone, three identified the wrong session, and five said they did not notice a difference. In their consensus statement on congenital adrenal hyperplasia, the Lawson Wilkins Pediatric Endocrine Society and European Society for Paediatric Endocrinology did not recommend increasing the glucocorticoid dose during psychological and emotional stress [48]. Therefore, although the topic is still open to discussion, it is important to state that young subjects should be advised not to take extra doses of hydrocortisone regularly (especially for day-to-day physical or psychological stressors), in order to minimize the long-term effects of chronic high-dose glucocorticoids. During hospitalization, major trauma, or surgery, intravenous hydrocortisone should be administered at a dosage of 50–100 mg/m^2/day divided into four doses (a bolus dose of 25 mg in neonates, infants, and preschool children, 50 mg in school-age children, and 100 mg in adults followed by three to four times the maintenance daily dose divided every 6 h) [101]. Hydrocortisone has mineralocorticoid activity at stress doses of 50 mg/m^2, hence mineralocorticoid supplementation is not required.

Surgical or trauma patients may receive rectal, intramuscular, or intravenous hydrocortisone. Intravenous bolus and subsequent dosage guidelines are as follows: for children younger than 3 years, 25 mg followed by 25–30 mg/day; for children 3–12 years of age, 50 mg followed by 50–60 mg/day; and for adolescents and adults, 100 mg followed by 100 mg/day [48, 101]. The most severe stresses, such as major surgery or sepsis, are often treated more aggressively, with dosages up to 100 mg/m^2 per day in divided doses every 6 h intravenously [99]. Although various glucocorticoid preparations could be used for stress dosing, hydrocortisone is the preferred agent because of its mineralocorticoid activity. Stress doses are administered for only 24–48 h unless the underlying illness is prolonged. Before general anesthesia and surgery, parenteral hydrocortisone is also recommended. A preoperative dose of 50 mg/m^2 30–60 min before induction of anesthesia can be administered intravenously or intramuscularly. A second dose of 50 mg/m^2 can then be administered as a constant infusion or as an intravenous bolus divided every 6 h over the next 24 h. Intravenous or oral stress doses may be continued until the patient has recovered [99].

For older adolescents and young adults, recently published guidelines [45] need to be followed during surgery, dental procedures, delivery, and invasive procedures, and are summarized in Table 5.

Role of Associated Hormonal Deficiencies or Treatment

Several studies have shown the role of multiple pituitary hormone deficiencies and especially of impaired thyroid function in defining glucocorticoid therapy. Adrenal crisis can develop after initiation of thyroid hormone replacement in subjects with hypothyroidism and with an accompanied unrecognized adrenal insufficiency. Although the underlying mechanisms are not fully understood, it has been hypothesized that patients with hypothyroidism have reduced cortisol requirements secondary to a reduced metabolic rate in the presence of untreated hypothyroidism [39,

Table 5 Treatment during surgery, dental procedures, delivery, and invasive procedures for fully grown youths and young adults (from Husebye et al.)

Procedure	Preoperative needs	Postoperative needs
Major surgery with long recovery time	100 mg hydrocortisone i.m. just before anesthesia	Continue 100 mg hydrocortisone i.m. every 6 h until able to eat and drink. Then double oral dose for 48 h, then taper to normal dose
Major surgery with rapid recovery	100 mg hydrocortisone i.m. just before anesthesia	Continue 100 mg hydrocortisone i.m. every 6 h for 24–48 h. Then double oral dose for 24–48 h, then taper to normal dose
Labor and vaginal birth	100 mg hydrocortisone i.m. at onset of labor	Double oral dose for 24–48 h after delivery, then taper to normal dose
Minor surgery and major dental surgery	100 mg hydrocortisone i.m. just before anesthesia	Double oral dose for 24 h, then return to normal dose
Invasive bowel procedures requiring laxatives	Hospital admission overnight with 100 mg hydrocortisone i.m. and fluid, repeat dose before start of procedure	Double oral dose for 24 h, then return to normal dose
Other invasive procedures	100 mg hydrocortisone i.m. just before start of procedure	Double oral dose for 24 h, then return to normal dose
Dental procedure	Extra morning dose 1 h before surgery	Double oral dose for 24 h, then return to normal dose
Minor procedure	Usually not required	Extra dose (e.g., 20 mg hydrocortisone) if symptoms are present

98]. Soon after thyroid hormone replacement therapy is started, the metabolic rate and cortisol requirements increase, resulting in an adrenal crisis. Similarly, cortisol metabolism is significantly increased in subjects with hyperthyroidism, thus resulting in an increased glucocorticoid requirement. Because of elevated cortisol clearance, it is suggested to increase cortisol replacement as much as twofold in individuals with hyperthyroidism and adrenal insufficiency [4].

Studies have shown that growth hormone treatment can affect cortisol levels. By inhibiting 11-β-HDS-1 activity in the liver, growth hormone treatment can result in decreased conversion of inactive cortisone to active cortisol [35]. Therefore, in subjects with secondary adrenal insufficiency requiring growth hormone therapy, signs and symptoms of adrenal insufficiency need to be monitored and glucocorticoid therapy increased accordingly. In addition, in children with anatomic abnormalities of the pituitary or stalk on magnetic resonance imaging, or with organic causes (e.g., cranial surgery, tumors, trauma) and/or multiple anterior pituitary hormone deficiencies, the hypothalamic–pituitary–adrenal axis should be evaluated. Similar considerations apply for children with cranial radiation, septo-optic dysplasia, autoimmune hypophysitis, PROP-1 deficiency, and head trauma [8, 15, 83]. If indicated, periodic reassessment of previously normal hypothalamic–pituitary–adrenal function should be considered in patients with organic hypopituitarism.

Hypothalamic–pituitary–adrenal function needs to be evaluated in children who receive medication able to affect cortisol biosynthesis, such as drugs that accelerate (i.e., phenytoin, barbiturates, and rifampin) [4, 99] or inhibit (i.e., aminoglutethimide, etomidate, ketoconazole, metyrapone, medroxyprogesterone, and megestrol) [27, 99] cortisol metabolism.

Lastly, but no less important, the hypothalamic–pituitary–adrenal axis should be explored in children and adolescents who have discontinued long-term glucocorticoid treatment. Chronic administration of synthetic glucocorticoids leads to feedback inhibition of endogenous cortisol secretion and may eventually induce adrenal insufficiency, with weakness, fatigue, or nausea. In these subjects, signs of adrenal insufficiency might particularly occur during stress after therapy is discontinued, due to an insufficient capacity of the adrenals to respond to stress. Recovery of the hypothalamic–pituitary–adrenal axis usually occurs within weeks after short-term (up to 3 months) therapy, but may occasionally take many months [40, 80, 95].

Pregnancy

Pregnancy and especially its related hormonal and metabolic changes represent a physiological condition requiring glucocorticoid adjustment in subjects. Owing to the effects of estrogen on liver, pregnancy is physiologically associated with a gradual and pronounced increase in corticosteroid-binding globulin production, which in turns results in increased levels of free cortisol levels, particularly during the last trimester. Additional factors such as the placental synthesis and release of biologically active CRH and ACTH, increased ACTH responsiveness, pituitary desensitization to cortisol feedback, and enhanced pituitary responses to corticotropin-releasing factors [62, 106] represent determinant contributors of the progressive free cortisol rise during pregnancy, up to twofold [1, 62, 106]. Thus, during pregnancy hydrocortisone doses might be increased by 50 % [4]. However, although physiological requirements increase during pregnancy, the need for hydrocortisone replacement dose adjustment during the last trimester is still debated. In single case reports, adrenal crisis due to insufficient dose adaptation during pregnancy has been observed. Therefore, we recommend close supervision and favor an increase in the glucocorticoid replacement dose by up to 50 % during the last trimester. In addition, a recent consensus statement in subjects with primary adrenal insufficiency recommended administering 100 mg of hydrocortisone intramuscularly at onset of labor, continuing with a double oral dose for 24–48 h after delivery and followed by rapid tapering [45].

Newer Formulations of Hydrocortisone

In some subjects treated with hydrocortisone, the replacement therapy often does not fully replicate the normal circadian pattern of cortisol secretion, thus significantly affecting disease control. Therefore, during the past few decades researchers attempted to overcome this issue by formulating new preparations of hydrocortisone, such as continuous subcutaneous infusion or modified-release hydrocortisone (MR-HC; Chronocort®), with promising preliminary results.

In a pilot study of adults, continuous subcutaneous hydrocortisone infusion was shown to properly restore the physiological circadian variation, resulting in a significant decrease of glucocorticoid daily doses [65]. Hydrocortisone infusion was not associated with major side effects and was linked to an improvement in subjective health status. Similarly, continuous subcutaneous infusion of hydrocortisone in a circadian pattern was able to achieve good disease control in a poorly controlled pubertal boy on high-dose oral treatment [17]. Results of phase II trials in the USA have shown that bedtime dosing of Chronocort® more closely mimics the physiological secretion pattern of cortisol and decreases morning 17-hydroxyprogesterone levels [113].

References

1. Allolio B, Hoffmann J, Linton EA, Winkelmann W, Kusche M, Schulte HM (1990) Diurnal salivary cortisol patterns during pregnancy and after delivery: relationship to plasma corticotrophin-releasing-hormone. Clin Endocrinol (Oxf) 33(2):279–289
2. Alonso N, Granada ML, Lucas A, Salinas I, Reverter J, Oriol A, Sanmarti A (2004) Evaluation of two replacement regimens in primary adrenal insufficiency patients. Effect on clinical symptoms, health-related quality of life and biochemical parameters. J Endocrinol Invest 27(5):449–454
3. Anderson JR, Goudie RB, Gray KG, Timbury GC (1957) Auto-antibodies in Addison's disease. Lancet 272(6979):1123–1124
4. Arlt W, Allolio B (2003) Adrenal insufficiency. Lancet 361(9372):1881–1893. doi:10.1016/S0140-6736(03)13492-7
5. Balsamo A, Baldazzi L, Menabo S, Cicognani A (2010) Impact of molecular genetics on congenital adrenal hyperplasia management. Sexual Dev Genet Mol Biol Evol Endocrinol Embryol Pathol Sex Determin Differ 4(4–5):233–248. doi:10.1159/000315959
6. Barbetta L, Dall'Asta C, Re T, Libe R, Costa E, Ambrosi B (2005) Comparison of different regimens of glucocorticoid replacement therapy in patients with hypoadrenalism. J Endocrinol Invest 28(7):632–637
7. Belgorosky A, Baquedano MS, Guercio G, Rivarola MA (2008) Adrenarche: postnatal adrenal zonation and hormonal and metabolic regulation. Horm Res 70(5):257–267. doi:10.1159/000157871
8. Benvenga S, Campenni A, Ruggeri RM, Trimarchi F (2000) Clinical review 113: hypopituitarism secondary to head trauma. J Clin Endocrinol Metab 85(4):1353–1361. doi:10.1210/jcem.85.4.6506
9. Bergendahl M, Iranmanesh A, Mulligan T, Veldhuis JD (2000) Impact of age on cortisol secretory dynamics basally and as driven by nutrient-withdrawal stress. J Clin Endocrinol Metab 85(6):2203–2214. doi:10.1210/jcem.85.6.6628
10. Betterle C, Dal Pra C, Mantero F, Zanchetta R (2002) Autoimmune adrenal insufficiency and autoimmune polyendocrine syndromes: autoantibodies, autoantigens, and their applicability in diagnosis and disease prediction. Endocr Rev 23(3):327–364. doi:10.1210/edrv.23.3.0466
11. Betterle C, Volpato M (1998) Adrenal and ovarian autoimmunity. Eur J Endocrinol/Eur Fed End Soc 138(1):16–25
12. Bonfiglio JJ, Inda C, Refojo D, Holsboer F, Arzt E, Silberstein S (2011) The corticotropin-releasing hormone network and the hypothalamic-pituitary-adrenal axis: molecular and cellular mechanisms involved. Neuroendocrinology 94(1):12–20. doi:10.1159/000328226

13. Boscaro M, Betterle C, Volpato M, Fallo F, Furmaniak J, Rees Smith B, Sonino N (1996) Hormonal responses during various phases of autoimmune adrenal failure: no evidence for 21-hydroxylase enzyme activity inhibition in vivo. J Clin Endocrinol Metab 81(8):2801–2804. doi:10.1210/jcem.81.8.8768833
14. Bose HS, Sugawara T, Strauss JF 3rd, Miller WL, International Congenital Lipoid Adrenal Hyperplasia C (1996) The pathophysiology and genetics of congenital lipoid adrenal hyperplasia. N Engl J Med 335(25):1870–1878. doi:10.1056/NEJM199612193352503
15. Bottner A, Keller E, Kratzsch J, Stobbe H, Weigel JF, Keller A, Hirsch W, Kiess W, Blum WF, Pfaffle RW (2004) PROP1 mutations cause progressive deterioration of anterior pituitary function including adrenal insufficiency: a longitudinal analysis. J Clin Endocrinol Metab 89(10):5256–5265. doi:10.1210/jc.2004-0661
16. Brandon DD, Isabelle LM, Samuels MH, Kendall JW, Loriaux DL (1999) Cortisol production rate measurement by stable isotope dilution using gas chromatography-negative ion chemical ionization mass spectrometry. Steroids 64(6):372–378
17. Bryan SM, Honour JW, Hindmarsh PC (2009) Management of altered hydrocortisone pharmacokinetics in a boy with congenital adrenal hyperplasia using a continuous subcutaneous hydrocortisone infusion. J Clin Endocrinol Metab 94(9):3477–3480. doi:10.1210/jc.2009-0630
18. Buttgereit F, Scheffold A (2002) Rapid glucocorticoid effects on immune cells. Steroids 67(6):529–534
19. Calogero AE, Gallucci WT, Chrousos GP, Gold PW (1988) Interaction between GABAergic neurotransmission and rat hypothalamic corticotropin-releasing hormone secretion in vitro. Brain Res 463(1):28–36
20. Chrousos GP (1998) Ultradian, circadian, and stress-related hypothalamic-pituitary-adrenal axis activity – a dynamic digital-to-analog modulation. Endocrinology 139(2):437–440. doi:10.1210/endo.139.2.5857
21. Chrousos GP (2000) The stress response and immune function: clinical implications. The 1999 Novera H. Spector Lecture. Ann N Y Acad Sci 917:38–67
22. Chrousos GP (2009) Stress and disorders of the stress system. Nat Rev Endocrinol 5(7):374–381. doi:10.1038/nrendo.2009.106
23. Chrousos GP, Gold PW (1992) The concepts of stress and stress system disorders. Overview of physical and behavioral homeostasis. JAMA 267(9):1244–1252
24. Chrousos GP, Kino T (2005) Intracellular glucocorticoid signaling: a formerly simple system turns stochastic. Sci STKE Signal Transduct Knowledge Environ (304):pe48. doi:10.1126/stke.3042005pe48
25. Cooper MS, Stewart PM (2003) Corticosteroid insufficiency in acutely ill patients. N Engl J Med 348(8):727–734. doi:10.1056/NEJMra020529
26. Coursin DB, Wood KE (2002) Corticosteroid supplementation for adrenal insufficiency. JAMA 287(2):236–240
27. den Brinker M, Joosten KF, Liem O, de Jong FH, Hop WC, Hazelzet JA, van Dijk M, Hokken-Koelega AC (2005) Adrenal insufficiency in meningococcal sepsis: bioavailable cortisol levels and impact of interleukin-6 levels and intubation with etomidate on adrenal function and mortality. J Clin Endocrinol Metab 90(9):5110–5117. doi:10.1210/jc.2005-1107
28. Esteban NV, Yergey AL (1990) Cortisol production rates measured by liquid chromatography/mass spectrometry. Steroids 55(4):152–158
29. Falorni A, Laureti S, De Bellis A, Zanchetta R, Tiberti C, Arnaldi G, Bini V, Beck-Peccoz P, Bizzarro A, Dotta F, Mantero F, Bellastella A, Betterle C, Santeusanio F, Group SIEAS (2004) Italian Addison network study: update of diagnostic criteria for the etiological classification of primary adrenal insufficiency. J Clin Endocrinol Metab 89(4):1598–1604. doi:10.1210/jc.2003-030954
30. Fragoso MC, Domenice S, Latronico AC, Martin RM, Pereira MA, Zerbini MC, Lucon AM, Mendonca BB (2003) Cushing's syndrome secondary to adrenocorticotropin-independent

macronodular adrenocortical hyperplasia due to activating mutations of GNAS1 gene. J Clin Endocrinol Metab 88(5):2147–2151. doi:10.1210/jc.2002-021362
31. Fuller RW (1992) The involvement of serotonin in regulation of pituitary-adrenocortical function. Front Neuroendocrinol 13(3):250–270
32. Funder JW (1997) Glucocorticoid and mineralocorticoid receptors: biology and clinical relevance. Annu Rev Med 48:231–240. doi:10.1146/annurev.med.48.1.231
33. Galon J, Franchimont D, Hiroi N, Frey G, Boettner A, Ehrhart-Bornstein M, O'Shea JJ, Chrousos GP, Bornstein SR (2002) Gene profiling reveals unknown enhancing and suppressive actions of glucocorticoids on immune cells. FASEB J Off Publ Fed Am Soc Exp Biol 16(1):61–71. doi:10.1096/fj.01-0245com
34. Gathercole LL, Lavery GG, Morgan SA, Cooper MS, Sinclair AJ, Tomlinson JW, Stewart PM (2013) 11beta-hydroxysteroid dehydrogenase 1: translational and therapeutic aspects. Endocr Rev 34(4):525–555. doi:10.1210/er.2012-1050
35. Giavoli C, Libe R, Corbetta S, Ferrante E, Lania A, Arosio M, Spada A, Beck-Peccoz P (2004) Effect of recombinant human growth hormone (GH) replacement on the hypothalamic-pituitary-adrenal axis in adult GH-deficient patients. J Clin Endocrinol Metab 89(11):5397–5401. doi:10.1210/jc.2004-1114
36. Gomez-Sanchez CE (2013) Adrenal dysfunction in critically ill patients. N Engl J Med 368(16):1547–1549. doi:10.1056/NEJMe1302305
37. Habib KE, Gold PW, Chrousos GP (2001) Neuroendocrinology of stress. Endocrinol Metab Clin North Am 30(3):695–728; vii–viii
38. Hartmann A, Veldhuis JD, Deuschle M, Standhardt H, Heuser I (1997) Twenty-four hour cortisol release profiles in patients with Alzheimer's and Parkinson's disease compared to normal controls: ultradian secretory pulsatility and diurnal variation. Neurobiol Aging 18(3):285–289
39. Havard CW, Saldanha VF, Bird R, Gardner R (1970) Adrenal function in hypothyroidism. Br Med J 1(5692):337–339
40. Henzen C, Suter A, Lerch E, Urbinelli R, Schorno XH, Briner VA (2000) Suppression and recovery of adrenal response after short-term, high-dose glucocorticoid treatment. Lancet 355(9203):542–545. doi:10.1016/S0140-6736(99)06290-X
41. Heuer H, Visser TJ (2009) Minireview: pathophysiological importance of thyroid hormone transporters. Endocrinology 150(3):1078–1083. doi:10.1210/en.2008-1518
42. Hiatt JR, Hiatt N (1997) The conquest of Addison's disease. Am J Surg 174(3):280–283
43. Howlett TA (1997) An assessment of optimal hydrocortisone replacement therapy. Clin Endocrinol (Oxf) 46(3):263–268
44. Hughes I (2002) Congenital adrenal hyperplasia: phenotype and genotype. J Pediatr Endocrinol Metabol JPEM 15(Suppl 5):1329–1340
45. Husebye ES, Allolio B, Arlt W, Badenhoop K, Bensing S, Betterle C, Falorni A, Gan EH, Hulting AL, Kasperlik-Zaluska A, Kampe O, Lovas K, Meyer G, Pearce SH (2014) Consensus statement on the diagnosis, treatment and follow-up of patients with primary adrenal insufficiency. J Intern Med 275(2):104–115. doi:10.1111/joim.12162
46. Invitti C, De Martin M, Delitala G, Veldhuis JD, Cavagnini F (1998) Altered morning and nighttime pulsatile corticotropin and cortisol release in polycystic ovary syndrome. Metabolism Clin Exp 47(2):143–148
47. Jansen M, Wit JM, van den Brande JL (1981) Reinstitution of mineralocorticoid therapy in congenital adrenal hyperplasia. Effects on control and growth. Acta Paediatr Scand 70(2):229–233
48. Joint LECAHWG (2002) Consensus statement on 21-hydroxylase deficiency from the Lawson Wilkins Pediatric Endocrine Society and the European Society for Paediatric Endocrinology. J Clin Endocrinol Metab 87(9):4048–4053. doi:10.1210/jc.2002-020611
49. Juszczak A, Ertorer ME, Grossman A (2013) The therapy of Cushing's disease in adults and children: an update. Horm Metab Res 45(2):109–117. doi:10.1055/s-0032-1330009
50. Kendall EC (1950) Cortisone. Ann Intern Med 33(4):787–796

51. Kerrigan JR, Veldhuis JD, Leyo SA, Iranmanesh A, Rogol AD (1993) Estimation of daily cortisol production and clearance rates in normal pubertal males by deconvolution analysis. J Clin Endocrinol Metab 76(6):1505–1510. doi:10.1210/jcem.76.6.8501158
52. Kino T, Chrousos GP (2001) Glucocorticoid and mineralocorticoid resistance/hypersensitivity syndromes. J Endocrinol 169(3):437–445
53. Kirk JM, Brain CE, Carson DJ, Hyde JC, Grant DB (1999) Cushing's syndrome caused by nodular adrenal hyperplasia in children with McCune-Albright syndrome. J Pediatr 134(6):789–792
54. Kong MF, Jeffcoate W (1994) Eighty-six cases of Addison's disease. Clin Endocrinol (Oxf) 41(6):757–761
55. Kraan GP, Dullaart RP, Pratt JJ, Wolthers BG, Drayer NM, De Bruin R (1998) The daily cortisol production reinvestigated in healthy men. The serum and urinary cortisol production rates are not significantly different. J Clin Endocrinol Metab 83(4):1247–1252. doi:10.1210/jcem.83.4.4694
56. Krone N, Braun A, Roscher AA, Knorr D, Schwarz HP (2000) Predicting phenotype in steroid 21-hydroxylase deficiency? Comprehensive genotyping in 155 unrelated, well defined patients from southern Germany. J Clin Endocrinol Metab 85(3):1059–1065. doi:10.1210/jcem.85.3.6441
57. Kyriazopoulou V (2007) Glucocorticoid replacement therapy in patients with Addison's disease. Expert Opin Pharmacother 8(6):725–729. doi:10.1517/14656566.8.6.725
58. Lamberts SW, Bruining HA, de Jong FH (1997) Corticosteroid therapy in severe illness. N Engl J Med 337(18):1285–1292. doi:10.1056/NEJM199710303371807
59. Laureti S, Falorni A, Santeusanio F (2003) Improvement of treatment of primary adrenal insufficiency by administration of cortisone acetate in three daily doses. J Endocrinol Invest 26(11):1071–1075
60. Levine A, Cohen D, Zadik Z (1994) Urinary free cortisol values in children under stress. J Pediatr 125(6 Pt 1):853–857
61. Linder BL, Esteban NV, Yergey AL, Winterer JC, Loriaux DL, Cassorla F (1990) Cortisol production rate in childhood and adolescence. J Pediatr 117(6):892–896
62. Lindsay JR, Nieman LK (2005) The hypothalamic-pituitary-adrenal axis in pregnancy: challenges in disease detection and treatment. Endocr Rev 26(6):775–799. doi:10.1210/er.2004-0025
63. Lodish M, Dunn SV, Sinaii N, Keil MF, Stratakis CA (2012) Recovery of the hypothalamic-pituitary-adrenal axis in children and adolescents after surgical cure of Cushing's disease. J Clin Endocrinol Metab 97(5):1483–1491. doi:10.1210/jc.2011-2325
64. Lodish MB, Sinaii N, Patronas N, Batista DL, Keil M, Samuel J, Moran J, Verma S, Popovic J, Stratakis CA (2009) Blood pressure in pediatric patients with Cushing syndrome. J Clin Endocrinol Metab 94(6):2002–2008. doi:10.1210/jc.2008-2694
65. Lovas K, Husebye ES (2007) Continuous subcutaneous hydrocortisone infusion in Addison's disease. Eur J Endocrinol/Eur Fed End Soc 157(1):109–112. doi:10.1530/EJE-07-0052
66. Lovas K, Husebye ES (2008) Replacement therapy for Addison's disease: recent developments. Expert Opin Investig Drugs 17(4):497–509. doi:10.1517/13543784.17.4.497
67. Magiakou MA, Mastorakos G, Oldfield EH, Gomez MT, Doppman JL, Cutler GB Jr, Nieman LK, Chrousos GP (1994) Cushing's syndrome in children and adolescents. Presentation, diagnosis, and therapy. N Engl J Med 331(10):629–636. doi:10.1056/NEJM199409083311002
68. Marik PE, Pastores SM, Annane D, Meduri GU, Sprung CL, Arlt W, Keh D, Briegel J, Beishuizen A, Dimopoulou I, Tsagarakis S, Singer M, Chrousos GP, Zaloga G, Bokhari F, Vogeser M, American College of Critical Care M (2008) Recommendations for the diagnosis and management of corticosteroid insufficiency in critically ill adult patients: consensus statements from an international task force by the American College of Critical Care Medicine. Crit Care Med 36(6):1937–1949. doi:10.1097/CCM.0b013e31817603ba
69. McEwen BS (2007) Physiology and neurobiology of stress and adaptation: central role of the brain. Physiol Rev 87(3):873–904. doi:10.1152/physrev.00041.2006

70. McEwen BS, Biron CA, Brunson KW, Bulloch K, Chambers WH, Dhabhar FS, Goldfarb RH, Kitson RP, Miller AH, Spencer RL, Weiss JM (1997) The role of adrenocorticoids as modulators of immune function in health and disease: neural, endocrine and immune interactions. Brain Res Brain Res Rev 23(1–2):79–133
71. Menon K, Lawson M (2007) Identification of adrenal insufficiency in pediatric critical illness. Pediatr Crit Care Med J Soc Crit Care Med World Fed Pediatr Intensive Crit Care Soc 8(3):276–278. doi:10.1097/01.PCC.0000262796.38637.15
72. Merke DP, Bornstein SR (2005) Congenital adrenal hyperplasia. Lancet 365(9477):2125–2136. doi:10.1016/S0140-6736(05)66736-0
73. Merke DP, Cho D, Calis KA, Keil MF, Chrousos GP (2001) Hydrocortisone suspension and hydrocortisone tablets are not bioequivalent in the treatment of children with congenital adrenal hyperplasia. J Clin Endocrinol Metab 86(1):441–445. doi:10.1210/jcem.86.1.7275
74. Migeon CJ, Green OC, Eckert JP (1963) Study of adrenocortical function in obesity. Metabolism Clin Exp 12:718–739
75. Miller WL (2007) StAR search – what we know about how the steroidogenic acute regulatory protein mediates mitochondrial cholesterol import. Mol Endocrinol 21(3):589–601. doi:10.1210/me.2006-0303
76. Mullis PE, Hindmarsh PC, Brook CG (1990) Sodium chloride supplement at diagnosis and during infancy in children with salt-losing 21-hydroxylase deficiency. Eur J Pediatr 150(1):22–25
77. Munck A, Guyre PM, Holbrook NJ (1984) Physiological functions of glucocorticoids in stress and their relation to pharmacological actions. Endocr Rev 5(1):25–44. doi:10.1210/edrv-5-1-25
78. Munck A, Naray-Fejes-Toth A (1992) The ups and downs of glucocorticoid physiology. Permissive and suppressive effects revisited. Mol Cell Endocrinol 90(1):C1–C4
79. Nerup J (1974) Addison's disease – a review of some clinical, pathological and immunological features. Dan Med Bull 21(6):201–217
80. Nicholson G, Burrin JM, Hall GM (1998) Peri-operative steroid supplementation. Anaesthesia 53(11):1091–1104
81. Nicolaides NC, Galata Z, Kino T, Chrousos GP, Charmandari E (2010) The human glucocorticoid receptor: molecular basis of biologic function. Steroids 75(1):1–12. doi:10.1016/j.steroids.2009.09.002
82. Nordenstrom A, Marcus C, Axelson M, Wedell A, Ritzen EM (1999) Failure of cortisone acetate treatment in congenital adrenal hyperplasia because of defective 11beta-hydroxysteroid dehydrogenase reductase activity. J Clin Endocrinol Metab 84(4):1210–1213. doi:10.1210/jcem.84.4.5584
83. Oberfield SE, Chin D, Uli N, David R, Sklar C (1997) Endocrine late effects of childhood cancers. J Pediatr 131(1 Pt 2):S37–S41
84. Oelkers W (1996) Adrenal insufficiency. N Engl J Med 335(16):1206–1212. doi:10.1056/NEJM199610173351607
85. Orth DN (1995) Cushing's syndrome. N Engl J Med 332(12):791–803. doi:10.1056/NEJM199503233321207
86. Payne AH, Hales DB (2004) Overview of steroidogenic enzymes in the pathway from cholesterol to active steroid hormones. Endocr Rev 25(6):947–970. doi:10.1210/er.2003-0030
87. Peacey SR, Guo CY, Robinson AM, Price A, Giles MA, Eastell R, Weetman AP (1997) Glucocorticoid replacement therapy: are patients over treated and does it matter? Clin Endocrinol (Oxf) 46(3):255–261
88. Ramakrishnan R, DuBois DC, Almon RR, Pyszczynski NA, Jusko WJ (2002) Pharmacodynamics and pharmacogenomics of methylprednisolone during 7-day infusions in rats. J Pharmacol Exp Ther 300(1):245–256
89. Reddy TE, Pauli F, Sprouse RO, Neff NF, Newberry KM, Garabedian MJ, Myers RM (2009) Genomic determination of the glucocorticoid response reveals unexpected mechanisms of gene regulation. Genome Res 19(12):2163–2171. doi:10.1101/gr.097022.109

90. Rhen T, Cidlowski JA (2005) Antiinflammatory action of glucocorticoids – new mechanisms for old drugs. N Engl J Med 353(16):1711–1723. doi:10.1056/NEJMra050541
91. Rivkees SA, Crawford JD (2000) Dexamethasone treatment of virilizing congenital adrenal hyperplasia: the ability to achieve normal growth. Pediatrics 106(4):767–773
92. Rubin RP (2007) A brief history of great discoveries in pharmacology: in celebration of the centennial anniversary of the founding of the American Society of Pharmacology and Experimental Therapeutics. Pharmacol Rev 59(4):289–359. doi:10.1124/pr.107.70102
93. Sapolsky RM, Romero LM, Munck AU (2000) How do glucocorticoids influence stress responses? Integrating permissive, suppressive, stimulatory, and preparative actions. Endocr Rev 21(1):55–89. doi:10.1210/edrv.21.1.0389
94. Sarnyai Z, Veldhuis JD, Mello NK, Mendelson JH, Eros-Sarnyai M, Mercer G, Gelles H, Kelly M (1995) The concordance of pulsatile ultradian release of adrenocorticotropin and cortisol in male rhesus monkeys. J Clin Endocrinol Metab 80(1):54–59. doi:10.1210/jcem.80.1.7829639
95. Schlaghecke R, Kornely E, Santen RT, Ridderskamp P (1992) The effect of long-term glucocorticoid therapy on pituitary-adrenal responses to exogenous corticotropin-releasing hormone. N Engl J Med 326(4):226–230. doi:10.1056/NEJM199201233260403
96. Seckl JR, Walker BR (2001) Minireview: 11beta-hydroxysteroid dehydrogenase type 1- a tissue-specific amplifier of glucocorticoid action. Endocrinology 142(4):1371–1376. doi:10.1210/endo.142.4.8114
97. Seckl JR, Walker BR (2004) 11beta-hydroxysteroid dehydrogenase type 1 as a modulator of glucocorticoid action: from metabolism to memory. Trends Endocrinol Metab TEM 15(9):418–424. doi:10.1016/j.tem.2004.09.007
98. Shaikh MG, Lewis P, Kirk JM (2004) Thyroxine unmasks Addison's disease. Acta Paediatr 93(12):1663–1665
99. Shulman DI, Palmert MR, Kemp SF, Lawson Wilkins D, Therapeutics C (2007) Adrenal insufficiency: still a cause of morbidity and death in childhood. Pediatrics 119(2):e484–e494. doi:10.1542/peds. 2006-1612
100. Silva Rdo C, Castro M, Kater CE, Cunha AA, Moraes AM, Alvarenga DB, Moreira AC, Elias LL (2004) Primary adrenal insufficiency in adults: 150 years after Addison. Arq Bras Endocrinol Metabol 48(5):724–738. doi:http://dx.doi.org/10.1590/S0004-27302004000500019
101. Speiser PW, Azziz R, Baskin LS, Ghizzoni L, Hensle TW, Merke DP, Meyer-Bahlburg HF, Miller WL, Montori VM, Oberfield SE, Ritzen M, White PC, Endocrine S (2010) Congenital adrenal hyperplasia due to steroid 21-hydroxylase deficiency: an Endocrine Society clinical practice guideline. J Clin Endocrinol Metab 95(9):4133–4160. doi:10.1210/jc.2009-2631
102. Spinner MW, Blizzard RM, Childs B (1968) Clinical and genetic heterogeneity in idiopathic Addison's disease and hypoparathyroidism. J Clin Endocrinol Metab 28(6):795–804. doi:10.1210/jcem-28-6-795
103. Stikkelbroeck NM, Hoefsloot LH, de Wijs IJ, Otten BJ, Hermus AR, Sistermans EA (2003) CYP21 gene mutation analysis in 198 patients with 21-hydroxylase deficiency in The Netherlands: six novel mutations and a specific cluster of four mutations. J Clin Endocrinol Metab 88(8):3852–3859. doi:10.1210/jc.2002-021681
104. Stratakis CA (2008) Cushing syndrome caused by adrenocortical tumors and hyperplasias (corticotropin- independent Cushing syndrome). Endocr Dev 13:117–132. doi:10.1159/000134829
105. Stratakis CA, Kirschner LS (1998) Clinical and genetic analysis of primary bilateral adrenal diseases (micro- and macronodular disease) leading to Cushing syndrome. Horm Metab Res 30(6–7):456–463. doi:10.1055/s-2007-978914
106. Suri D, Moran J, Hibbard JU, Kasza K, Weiss RE (2006) Assessment of adrenal reserve in pregnancy: defining the normal response to the adrenocorticotropin stimulation test. J Clin Endocrinol Metab 91(10):3866–3872. doi:10.1210/jc.2006-1049

107. Thompson EB, Tomkins GM, Curran JF (1966) Induction of tyrosine alpha-ketoglutarate transaminase by steroid hormones in a newly established tissue culture cell line. Proc Natl Acad Sci U S A 56(1):296–303
108. Tomlinson JW, Walker EA, Bujalska IJ, Draper N, Lavery GG, Cooper MS, Hewison M, Stewart PM (2004) 11beta-hydroxysteroid dehydrogenase type 1: a tissue-specific regulator of glucocorticoid response. Endocr Rev 25(5):831–866. doi:10.1210/er.2003-0031
109. Tsigos C, Chrousos GP (1996) Differential diagnosis and management of Cushing's syndrome. Annu Rev Med 47:443–461. doi:10.1146/annurev.med.47.1.443
110. Turnbull AV, Rivier CL (1999) Regulation of the hypothalamic-pituitary-adrenal axis by cytokines: actions and mechanisms of action. Physiol Rev 79(1):1–71
111. Valenzuela GA, Smalley WE, Schain DC, Vance ML, McCallum RW (1987) Reversibility of gastric dysmotility in cortisol deficiency. Am J Gastroenterol 82(10):1066–1068
112. Veldhuis JD (1997) How does one get at glandular secretion, when only hormone concentrations are measured? Clin Endocrinol (Oxf) 46(4):397–400
113. Verma S, Vanryzin C, Sinaii N, Kim MS, Nieman LK, Ravindran S, Calis KA, Arlt W, Ross RJ, Merke DP (2010) A pharmacokinetic and pharmacodynamic study of delayed- and extended-release hydrocortisone (Chronocort) vs. conventional hydrocortisone (Cortef) in the treatment of congenital adrenal hyperplasia. Clin Endocrinol (Oxf) 72(4):441–447. doi:10.1111/j.1365-2265.2009.03636.x
114. Weise M, Drinkard B, Mehlinger SL, Holzer SM, Eisenhofer G, Charmandari E, Chrousos GP, Merke DP (2004) Stress dose of hydrocortisone is not beneficial in patients with classic congenital adrenal hyperplasia undergoing short-term, high-intensity exercise. J Clin Endocrinol Metab 89(8):3679–3684. doi:10.1210/jc.2003-032051
115. White PC, Speiser PW (2000) Congenital adrenal hyperplasia due to 21-hydroxylase deficiency. Endocr Rev 21(3):245–291. doi:10.1210/edrv.21.3.0398
116. Windle RJ, Wood SA, Shanks N, Lightman SL, Ingram CD (1998) Ultradian rhythm of basal corticosterone release in the female rat: dynamic interaction with the response to acute stress. Endocrinology 139(2):443–450. doi:10.1210/endo.139.2.5721
117. Winqvist O, Karlsson FA, Kampe O (1992) 21-hydroxylase, a major autoantigen in idiopathic Addison's disease. Lancet 339(8809):1559–1562
118. Young EA, Abelson J, Lightman SL (2004) Cortisol pulsatility and its role in stress regulation and health. Front Neuroendocrinol 25(2):69–76. doi:10.1016/j.yfrne.2004.07.001

Systemic Corticosteroids in Respiratory Diseases in Children

Chiara Caparrelli, Claudia Calogero, and Enrico Lombardi

Introduction

Corticosteroids are anti-inflammatory drugs that have been used for the treatment of respiratory diseases for many decades. Despite their long use, the role of steroids in several respiratory conditions is still highly debated.

Corticosteroids inhibit the release of several cytokines and proinflammatory mediators and have a direct action on certain inflammatory cells. They accelerate the apoptosis of eosinophils and, although they are not effective in inhibiting the release of mediators from mast cells, after long-term treatment corticosteroids reduce the number of mucosal mast cells in the airways. Furthermore, glucocorticoids inhibit the increase of vascular permeability caused by inflammatory mediators with a direct effect on postcapillary venules of the respiratory epithelium and reduce the production of mucus in the airways.

Asthma

One of the most common respiratory diseases in children is asthma, which is a chronic inflammatory disease of the lower airways characterized by bronchial obstruction, usually reversible spontaneously or in response to therapy, and bronchial hyperreactivity. Systemic corticosteroids are rarely necessary in the long-term treatment of asthma in children. They should be considered only in patients with severe asthma and used at the lowest dose necessary to control symptoms. In

C. Caparrelli • C. Calogero • E. Lombardi (✉)
Paediatric Pulmonary Unit, "Anna Meyer" Paediatric University-Hospital, Florence, Italy
e-mail: e.lombardi@meyer.it

R. Cimaz (ed.), *Systemic Corticosteroids for Inflammatory Disorders in Pediatrics*, DOI 10.1007/978-3-319-16056-6_12

children with uncontrolled asthma needing systemic steroids, other drugs can be considered, even if most treatments are unlicensed and studies of these treatments are few. An exception is omalizumab, an anti-immunoglobulin E (IgE) monoclonal antibody. The most recent asthma guidelines, such as the update of the National Institute for Health and Care Excellence guidance in 2013, the International Consensus on Asthma guidelines, and the update of the Global Initiative on Asthma guidelines in 2014, recommend omalizumab as add-on therapy in adults and children over 6 years of age with uncontrolled IgE-mediated asthma who require frequent use of oral corticosteroids [1, 2].

Many studies have shown that systemic corticosteroids are useful in the treatment of acute asthma. In fact, they improve symptoms, oxygenation, and pulmonary function and reduce hospital admissions [3, 4]. Some studies showed that systemic steroids are more effective in patients with severe asthma and that they may not be useful for treating mild attacks of asthma that respond well to bronchodilators, except for children who have been hospitalized or previously intubated or who are already treated with oral steroids.

Oral and parenteral corticosteroids seem to have the same effects in most patients, and there are no significant differences of efficacy between different systemic steroids administered in equipotent doses. In general, the dose of systemic corticosteroids given is 1–2 mg/kg of prednisone in one or two doses, and the duration of treatment is usually 3–10 days depending on the severity of the attack and the clinical response [5].

Preschool Wheezing

Oral steroids are widely used to treat preschool children with wheezing, but their efficacy is controversial. Preschool wheezing is a common condition that usually regresses in the first 6 years of life. Three randomized control trials (RCTs) showed a positive but not significant effect of systemic steroids in children with wheezing admitted to emergency departments [6, 7]. A recent study has shown that oral prednisolone given for 5 days at the beginning of an attack of viral wheeze in preschool children has no benefits [8]. A more recent trial reported that in preschool children with mild or moderate wheeze admitted to hospital, oral prednisolone is not superior to placebo [9].

Rhinovirus infection is an important risk factor for recurrent wheezing in preschool children. A recent RCT reported that oral prednisolone is not superior to placebo in preventing the recurrence of wheezing in children whose first wheezing episode was caused by rhinovirus. However, the same study reported that oral prednisolone might be useful in a subgroup of children with high viral load [10].

In conclusion, oral steroids cannot be recommended in all cases of viral wheeze. They should be given only to preschool children admitted to hospital who are not responding to bronchodilators or with risk factors for asthma such as atopic eczema or a family history of asthma [11, 12].

Bronchiolitis

Another common respiratory disease in children is bronchiolitis, which is the most common lower respiratory tract infection in the first year of life. Oxygen supplementation and other supportive treatment such as feeding, hydration, and nasal suctioning are the main therapy for bronchiolitis [13]. Systematic reviews and meta-analyses of RCTs involving 1,200 children with viral bronchiolitis have not provided sufficient evidence to support the use of steroids in this illness [14, 15]. The recent guidelines of the American Academy of Pediatrics state that systemic corticosteroids should not be used routinely in the treatment of bronchiolitis [15].

Community-Acquired Pneumonia

Systemic corticosteroids are also used in community-acquired pneumonia (CAP), another frequent disease of the lower airways in children. The benefits of corticosteroids in the treatment of CAP in adults are not clear and even fewer data are available on the use of steroids in children with CAP. A recent prospective observational study reported that treatment with corticosteroids in CAP in adults is not associated with lower mortality and does not change the length of hospital stay or the readmission rate. A randomized double-blinded clinical trial with 213 adults concluded that systemic prednisolone has no positive effects in patients hospitalized with CAP [16]. A recent study reported that systemic steroids in adult patients with CAP do not influence the mortality rate or clinical course of the disease, but seem to prolong the duration of hospitalization [17].

A further study investigated a 5-day course of methylprednisolone therapy in 29 children with severe CAP treated with imipenem. This group was compared with 30 patients treated with imipenem and placebo [18]. The authors reported that methylprednisolone significantly reduced the length of hospital stay as well as the number of severe complications and of surgical interventions [18].

A multicenter retrospective study of 20,703 children with CAP showed that systemic corticosteroids are useful only in patients with acute wheezing, in whom they reduce the duration of hospitalization, whereas in those with CAP without wheezing, systemic steroids are associated with a longer hospital stay and a greater rate of readmission [19].

Thus, currently systemic corticosteroids cannot be recommended as adjunctive treatment in children with CAP [20], but further large RCTs are necessary to investigate the efficacy and safety of systemic corticosteroids in these children.

Bronchopulmonary Dysplasia

Another disease of the lower airways in children is bronchopulmonary dysplasia (BPD), an alteration of lung development as a result of multiple insults to the lung of the fetus and the premature newborn. An important role in the pathogenesis of BPD is played by persistent lung inflammation, and corticosteroids have been administered widely in preterm infants with respiratory failure. There are many studies in which both systemic and inhaled corticosteroids have been used for the treatment and prevention of BPD. A Cochrane Review of 28 trials showed that systemic steroids administered in the first week of life facilitate extubation and decrease the incidence of BPD, but cause significant adverse effects such as gastrointestinal hemorrhage, bowel perforation, cardiomyopathy, and cerebral palsy [21]. Another Cochrane meta-analysis revealed that the use of steroids after the first 7 days is associated with a decreased risk of BPD and accelerated weaning from oxygen and mechanical ventilation with no increase in long-term adverse effects such as cerebral palsy [21, 22]. The European Association of Perinatal Medicine, the American Academy of Pediatrics, and the Canadian Pediatric Society stated there is no sufficient evidence to recommend routine use of steroids in preterm infants after the first week of life; however, a short course of dexamethasone can be considered in patients with BPD in whom weaning from mechanical ventilation and oxygen therapy is difficult or whose respiratory conditions are quickly worsening [21].

Allergic Bronchopulmonary Aspergillosis

Systemic corticosteroids, together with antifungal drugs, are the mainstay of therapy for allergic bronchopulmonary aspergillosis, which occurs often in patients with cystic fibrosis (CF). Several studies reported that systemic steroids in this condition decrease serum IgE levels and total eosinophil count and improve clinical symptoms and lung function. Oral corticosteroids are useful in allergic bronchopulmonary aspergillosis, but the adverse effects of a long-term treatment have led to a search for safer regimens. Some studies showed that monthly high doses of intravenous methylprednisolone led to improved clinical conditions and laboratory parameters with fewer side effects compared with oral steroids [23, 24]. Moreover, there are case reports that omalizumab may have beneficial effects in allergic bronchopulmonary aspergillosis, but RCTs in children are needed.

Cystic Fibrosis

The use of corticosteroids has also been investigated in the treatment of acute exacerbations in patients with CF. In a study of children with CF hospitalized for severe respiratory distress, the clinical conditions of the patients were improved by the administration of a high dose of methylprednisolone intravenously for 3 days; the authors concluded that this therapy could be an effective treatment for children with uncontrolled pulmonary exacerbations [25].

Given the role of lung inflammation in the pathogenesis of CF, systemic steroids have also been studied as long-term therapy in patients with this disease. A recent Cochrane Review identified three RCTs on oral corticosteroids given for more than 30 days in patients with CF. The authors concluded that long-term use of oral steroids at prednisolone-equivalent doses of 1–2 mg/kg on alternate days seemed to reduce the progression of lung disease, although often at the cost of adverse effects such as cataracts and growth retardation. Hence, long-term use of systemic steroids in patients with CF is not recommended [26].

Primary Ciliary Dyskinesia and Interstitial Lung Disease

Another disease of the lower airways characterized by lung inflammation and frequent infections is primary ciliary dyskinesia, which is defined as a group of congenital pathological conditions due to the abnormal structure and/or function of cilia, with altered mucociliary transport leading to several respiratory disorders.

There are no RCTs on the use of corticosteroids in this condition, and therefore indications are often based on expert opinion or are extrapolated from evidence available from CF studies. Inhaled or oral steroids together with bronchodilators are only prescribed if the child is thought to also have airflow obstruction [27]. Systemic corticosteroids are used for many interstitial lung diseases including surfactant protein deficiencies but there are no controlled trials in children; treatment is based on uncontrolled studies, case reports, and observations [28].

Bronchiolitis Obliterans

Another rare but severe chronic lung disease in children is bronchiolitis obliterans (BO). The most common presentation is the postinfectious variant, related to a viral lower respiratory tract infection in the first years of life [29]. BO is characterized by inflammation and fibrosis of bronchioli resulting in narrowing and obliteration of the small airways. There are few RCTs focusing on treatment of BO in children, and therapeutic decisions are often based on empirical evidence [29]. Inhaled corticosteroids are widely used in patients with BO; oral steroids are used during respiratory obstructive exacerbations for variable periods or in patients with severe oxygen-dependent BO [29]. Currently, the use of systemic corticosteroids in the treatment of BO is controversial. A recent study suggested that intravenous pulse corticosteroids could be a useful and relatively safe treatment option in children with BO, with fewer adverse effects compared with continuous therapy with oral steroids. New prospective controlled trials are required to confirm this therapeutic regimen [30].

Croup

A common disease of the upper airways in which corticosteroids are widely used is croup, characterized by acute obstruction. Viral croup mainly affects children between 6 months and 6 years of age. Many RCTs have demonstrated significant benefits of corticosteroids in patients with croup; systemic or nebulized steroids decrease the need for other drugs, the duration of hospital stay, and the need for intubation [31].

Conclusion

Systemic corticosteroids are used in various respiratory diseases in children. However, the role of systemic steroids in children is limited by their side effects. Physicians must always weigh the benefits against the potential adverse effects when they decide to use corticosteroids in children.

Steroids are useful in the treatment of acute asthma and croup. In conditions such as bronchiolitis, preschool wheezing, bronchopulmonary dysplasia, and community-acquired pneumonia, their benefits are uncertain and they cannot be recommended routinely. In other rare respiratory diseases, systemic corticosteroids are used despite the lack of scientific evidence of their benefits.

References

1. Normansell R, Walker S, Milan SJ, Walters EH, Nair P (2014) Omalizumab for asthma in adults and children. Cochrane Database Syst Rev (1):CD003559
2. D'Amato G, Stanzola A, Sanduzzi A, Liccardi G, Salzillo A, Vitale C, Molino A, Vatrella A, D'Amato M (2014) Treating severe allergic asthma with anti-IgE monoclonal antibody (omalizumab): a review. Multidiscip Respir Med 9(1):23
3. Rowe BH, Spooner C, Ducharme FM, Bretzlaff JA, Bota GW (2001) Early emergency department treatment of acute asthma with systemic corticosteroids. Cochrane Database Syst Rev (1):CD002178

4. Hendeles L (2003) Selecting a systemic corticosteroid for acute asthma in young children. J Pediatr 142:S40–S44
5. Jones MA, Wagener JS (2001) Managing acute pediatric asthma: keeping it short. J Pediatr 139:3–5
6. Tal A, Levy N, Bearman JE (1990) Methylprednisolone therapy for acute asthma in infants and toddlers: a controlled clinical trial. Pediatrics 86:350–356
7. Csonka P, Kaila M, Laippala P, Iso-Mustaja M, Vesikari T, Ashborn P (2003) Oral prednisolone in the acute management of children age 6 to 35 months with viral respiratory infection-induced lower airway disease: a randomized, placebo-controlled trial. J Pediatr 143:725–730
8. Oommen A, Lambert PC, Grigg J (2003) Efficacy of a short course of parent-initiated oral prednisolone for viral wheeze in children aged 1–5 years: randomized controlled trial. Lancet 362:1433–1438
9. Panickar J, Lakhanpaul M, Lambert PC, Kenia P, Stephenson T, Smyth A, Grigg J (2009) Oral prednisolone for preschool children with acute virus-induced wheezing. N Engl J Med 360:329–338
10. Jartti T, Nieminen R, Vuorinen T, Lehtinen P, Vahlberg T, Gern J, Camargo CA Jr, Ruuskanen O (2015) Short- and long-term efficacy of prednisolone for first acute rhinovirus-induced wheezing episode. J Allergy Clin Immunol 135:691–698
11. Vuillermin PJ, Robertson CF, South M (2007) Parent-initiated oral corticosteroid therapy for intermittent wheezing illnesses in children: systemic review. J Paediatr Child Health 43(6): 438–442
12. Vuillermin P, South M, Robertson C (2006) Parent-initiated oral corticosteroid therapy for intermittent wheezing illnesses in children. Cochrane Database Syst Rev (3):CD005311
13. Da Dalt L, Bressan S, Martinolli F, Perilongo G, Baraldi E (2013) Treatment of bronchiolitis: state of the art. Early Hum Dev 89(Suppl 1):S31–S36
14. Fernandes RM, Bialy LM, Vandermeer B, Tjosvold L, Plint AC, Patel H, Johnson DW, Klassen TP, Hartling L (2010) Glucocorticoids for acute viral bronchiolitis in infants and young children. Cochrane Database Syst Rev (10):CD004878
15. American Academy of Pediatrics. Subcommittee on Diagnosis and Management of Bronchiolitis (2006) Diagnosis and management of bronchiolitis. Pediatrics 118:1774–1793
16. Snijders D, Daniels JM, De Graaff CS, Van Der Werf TS, Boersma WG (2010) Efficacy of corticosteroids in community-acquired pneumonia randomized double-blinded clinical trial. Am J Respir Crit Care Med 181(9):975–982
17. Polverino E, Cilloniz C, Dambrava P, Gabarrus A, Ferrer M, Agusti C, Prina E, Montull B, Menedez R, Niederman MS (2013) Systemic corticosteroids for community-acquired pneumonia: reasons for use and lack of benefit on outcome. Respirology 18(2):263–271
18. Nagy B, Gaspar I, Papp A, Bene Z, Nagy B Jr, Voko Z, Balla G (2013) Efficacy of methylprednisolone in children with severe community acquired pneumonia. Pediatr Pulmonol 48(2): 168–175
19. Weiss AK, Hall M, Lee GE, Kronman MP, Sheffler-Collins S, Shah SS (2011) Adjunct corticosteroids in children hospitalized with community acquired pneumonia. Pediatrics 127(2):e255–e263
20. Salluh J, Povoa P, Soares M, Castro-Faria-Neto HC, Bozza FA, Bozza PT (2008) The role of corticosteroids in severe community-acquired pneumonia: a systematic review. Crit Care 12(3):R76
21. Ghanta S, Leeman KT, Christou H (2013) An update on pharmacologic approaches to bronchopulmonary dysplasia. Semin Perinatol 37(2):115–123
22. Jain D, Bancalani E (2014) Bronchopulmonary dysplasia: clinical perspective. Birth Defects Res A Clin Mol Teratol 100(3):134–144
23. Thomson JM, Wesley A, Byrnes CA, Nixon GM (2006) Pulse intravenous methylprednisolone for resistant allergic bronchopulmonary aspergillosis in cystic fibrosis. Pediatr Pulmonol 41(2):164–170

24. Cohen-Cymberknoh M, Blau H, Shoseyov D, Mei-Zahav M, Efrati O, Armoni S, Kerem E (2009) Intravenous monthly pulse methylprednisolone treatment for ABPA in patients with cystic fibrosis. J Cyst Fibros 8(4):253–257
25. Ghdifan S, Couderc L, Michelet I, Leguillon C, Masseline B, Marguet C (2010) Bolus methylprednisolone efficacy for uncontrolled exacerbation of cystic fibrosis in children. Pediatrics 125(5):e1259–e1264
26. Cheng K, Ashby D, Smyth RL (2013) Oral steroids for long-term use in cystic fibrosis. Cochrane Database Syst Rev (6):CD000407
27. Pifferi M, Di Cicco M, Piras M, Cangiotti AM, Saggese G (2013) Up to date on primary ciliary dyskinesia in children. Early Hum Dev 89(Suppl 3):S45–S48
28. Kurland G, Deterding RR, Hagood JS, Young LR, Brody AS, Castile RG, Dell S, Fan LL, Hamvas A, Hilman BC, Langston C, Nogee LM, Redding GJ, American Thoracic Society Committee on Childhood Interstitial Lung Disease (chILD) and the chILD Research Network (2013) An official American Thoracic Society clinical practice guideline: classification, evaluation, and management of childhood interstitial lung disease in infancy. Am J Respir Crit Care Med 188(3):376–394
29. Fischer GB, Sarria EE, Mattiello R, Mocelin HT, Castro-Rodriguez JA (2010) Post infectious bronchiolitis obliterans in children. Paediatr Respir Rev 11(4):233–239
30. Tomikawa SO, Adde FV, da Silva Filho LV, Leone C, Rodrigues JC (2014) Follow-up on pediatric patients with bronchiolitis obliterans treated with corticosteroid pulse therapy. Orphanet J Rare Dis 9:128
31. De Benedictis FM, Bush A (2012) Corticosteroids in respiratory diseases in children. Am J Respir Crit Care Med 185(1):12–23

Corticosteroids in Pediatric Nephrology

Kjell Tullus

Nephrotic Syndrome

Nephrotic syndrome (NS) is not a disease but a syndrome characterized by the combination of massive proteinuria, low serum albumin, and edema [1]. There are several potential causes of NS, but so-called idiopathic NS is by far the most common in pediatrics. The typical presentation is a young child, 2–4 years old, who without any other symptoms starts to show edema. This typically begins around the eyes and occurs early in the morning. Often, it is initially misdiagnosed as allergic eye symptoms. The edema then develops further with swelling of the legs, genitalia, and ascites [1].

The cause of idiopathic NS is in most cases not known. There are no clinical or laboratory signs of any other disease or any inflammation [1]. If the children do not display any atypical features, they are started on treatment with prednisolone without further investigation. The dose used is 2 mg/kg or 60 mg/m^2 (maximum dose, 60 mg).

The majority of children with NS respond to this treatment within 4 weeks, normally already after a few weeks. The proteinuria disappears totally, the serum albumin rises to normal concentrations, and the edema goes away. These children are said to have steroid-sensitive NS [1].

Different steroid regimens have been used. A classic regimen was devised by the International Study for Kidney Diseases in Childhood (ISKDC); they recommended a high dose for 4 weeks and then another 4 weeks of 1.5 mg/kg or 40 mg/m^2 on alternate days [2]. Other regimens have advocated longer initial treatment. A meta-analysis showed that longer treatment courses seemed to give longer relapse-free

K. Tullus, MD, PhD, FRCPCH
Nephrology, Great Ormond Street Hospital for Children,
Great Ormond Street, London WC1N 3JH, UK
e-mail: Kjell.Tullus@gosh.nhs.uk

R. Cimaz (ed.), *Systemic Corticosteroids for Inflammatory Disorders in Pediatrics*, DOI 10.1007/978-3-319-16056-6_13

intervals [3]. It was recommended that children should initially be given at least 3 months of prednisolone with possibly fewer relapses with treatment extending up to 7 months. This obviously contrasts markedly with the need to keep the dose as low and as short as possible to prevent accumulating toxicity.

However, a more recent study could not confirm that extending the prednisolone treatment reduced relapses [4]. Further trials on this topic are ongoing and controversies still exist on how much and for how long children with first-time NS should be treated [5].

Children with steroid-sensitive NS can develop different clinical courses: A majority will continue to have occasional relapses of NS and need further treatment that they normally will respond to well. Other groups of children will develop frequently relapsing NS or steroid-dependent NS, while yet another group will not respond to the steroid treatment and become steroid resistant (SRNS).

The prognosis of NS in children is generally very good. Most children will, after a number of relapses, grow out of their problem; this often happens during puberty. A majority of children will at that time have preserved and normal kidney function. The major long-term problem for this group of children is steroid toxicity. Many are left with obesity, striae, and other problems.

The mechanism of action of steroids in NS is totally unknown; an immune-mediated disease is generally suspected but there are no clinical or laboratory signs supporting this theory. It is, however, further supported by the fact that all other drugs that can be used in these children during later stages are also highly active immune-modulating agents.

Frequently Relapsing or Steroid-Dependent Nephrotic Syndrome

Most children with NS experience relapses that need treatment with prednisolone. This treatment is normally given as a full dose of 60 mg/m^2 until the child has been free of protein in the urine for 3 days and then 40 mg/m^2 every other day for a further 4 weeks. This is normally not a major problem if the children respond reasonably quickly to the treatment and the dose can thus be rapidly changed to an alternate-day regimen. The steroid toxicity can be managed in most of these cases. Some 30 % of children will, however, have frequent relapses resulting in many courses of prednisolone every year. These children are at high risk of developing intolerable steroid toxicity. They are often treated with alternate-day steroids at as low a dose as possible to keep them in remission. The alternate-day treatment was shown to be more successful than treatment during 3 consecutive days per week [6]. An alternate-day dose of up to 1 mg/kg did not have any long-term side effects on children's growth [7]. However, treatment with other immunosuppressive drugs is often needed to achieve the aim of minimizing the number of relapses and of full steroid courses.

A further somewhat overlapping group of children will develop steroid-dependent NS. They relapse while still on, or immediately after, a weaning dose of the drug. This can often be managed by keeping the child on an alternate-day dose that is low enough to keep them well but that does not have any discernible side effects [6, 7]. Many of these children will also need treatment with another drug to reduce their tendency to relapse.

Steroid-Resistant Nephrotic Syndrome

A small group of children with NS do not respond to the initial dose of prednisolone; they are defined as having steroid-resistant NS (SRNS) [1]. A common definition is there is no reduction in urinary losses of protein despite a 4-week course of prednisolone. Three pulses of intravenous methylprednisolone are often given to ensure the child has received the drug. In some cases it is suspected that the absorption of the drug has been inadequate owing to the often-occurring massive edema including intestinal edema. Further treatment protocols of SRNS usually include several doses of methylprednisolone [8, 9].

Patients with SRNS are in a far more difficult subgroup of NS than those who respond to steroids. They will need a kidney biopsy. The two most common biopsy diagnoses are minimal-change nephropathy (i.e., nothing significant is seen) and focal and segmental glomerulosclerosis. Children with focal and segmental glomerulosclerosis have a much more severe disease that often leads to end-stage renal disease requiring renal transplantation. Many of these children unfortunately have disease recurrence after the transplant, which can lead to rapid loss of the transplanted kidney [10].

A number of other immunosuppressive drugs are used in these children to try to achieve remission and to prevent the development of renal failure. This treatment can sometimes convert the condition of the children into being steroid sensitive.

Glomerulonephritis

Glomerulonephritis (GN) is a far less common disease in children compared with adult patients. The most common forms of GN that I will discuss here are postinfectious glomerulonephritis, systemic lupus erythematosus nephritis, Henoch–Schönlein purpura nephritis, and IgA nephropathy. I will omit other very uncommon forms of GN in childhood, such as membranoproliferative GN and membranous GN.

Postinfectious Glomerulonephritis

The most common form of postinfectious GN is poststreptococcal GN. These children typically present with hematuria, often macroscopic, mildly impaired kidney function, and somewhat raised blood pressure 1–2 weeks after a streptococcal infection [11]. The diagnosis is strengthened by the confirmation of the streptococcal infection, by the presence of rising streptococcal antibodies in serum, or a positive throat culture. Patients develop reduced complement C3 and C4 levels in blood, which should normalize within a few months.

Poststreptococcal GN is a self-limiting disease that should heal without any long-term sequelae [11]. Treatment with steroids is thus not needed in a vast majority of cases. A small minority will develop a rapidly progressing GN where the biopsy will show crescentic nephritis. These rare children might benefit from treatment with steroids (see next section).

Systemic Lupus Erythematosus Nephritis

Lupus nephritis is the most common severe nephritis in childhood. Its onset is mainly in prepubertal or pubertal girls who develop severe systemic symptoms over the course of a few weeks with fatigue, loss of appetite, weight loss, joint pain, and rash (typically malar). More than 50 % of children with lupus will develop nephritis characterized by microscopic hematuria and proteinuria and some impairment of the kidney function [12]. Many present with overt nephrotic syndrome with massive proteinuria, low serum albumin, and edema.

All these children should have a kidney biopsy to classify the degree of kidney involvement from Class I to V, and those with Class III–V nephritis should receive treatment focusing on the nephritis [13].

Treatment of lupus nephritis is generally done in two phases, induction and maintenance treatment, and steroids have always played a major role in both. Treatment of lupus nephritis is normally initiated with three infusions of high-dose methylprednisolone and then continued with a high dose of oral prednisolone; 2 mg/kg/day capped at 60 mg/day [13].

No consensus exists on how quickly to wean the steroid dose or on how low the dose should be during the maintenance phase. Some centers continue daily steroids at doses around 15 mg/day, while others aim for alternate-day dosing, and yet other centers try to stop the prednisolone when the child is well. Aggressive treatment with other immunosuppressive drugs, such as mycophenolate mofetil, cyclophosphamide, azathioprine, and rituximab, is essential so as to use as few steroids as possible [14].

Severe side effects from steroids are clearly a major problem for children and young people with lupus. Because of this, a relative steroid-free induction treatment of lupus nephritis has been attempted in adult patients with seemingly good results. Treatment started with three pulses of methylprednisolone together with two infusions of the CD20 antibody rituximab and oral mycophenolate mofetil [15]. No further steroid treatment was given. A randomized trial of this regimen is now underway including both adults and children.

This author strongly agrees that steroid side effects are a major clinical problem in children with lupus but would still caution against adopting the steroid-free regimen in children until more data have been generated. There is, however, a strong reason to always aim at steroid doses that are as low as possible in these children.

Henoch–Schönlein Purpura Nephritis

Henoch–Schönlein purpura (HSP) is an acute vasculitis that is relatively common in children. It typically includes a marked purpuric rash on the lower parts of the body, marked abdominal pain due to intestinal vasculitis, marked swelling and pain around the joints in the lower part of the body, and acute glomerulonephritis [16, 17]. Some children have all these features but many only experience some. HSP is self-limiting in the large majority of children who thus do not need any treatment. It can, however, have a relapsing and remitting course lasting several weeks. The disease is sometimes quite severe and treatment with steroids has been tried. However, it has not been shown to be beneficial except in cases with severe abdominal pain where a short course can be warranted [16].

A small minority of these children can develop a severe acute GN that shows a crescentic GN on biopsy. They should have the same treatment as that for rapidly progressing GN. A small percentage of children with HSP nephritis do not recover from their proteinuria and hematuria, and a chronic low-grade GN develops. This has biopsy features similar to IgA nephropathy [18] and these children should most likely be treated as patients with IgA nephropathy.

A course of 14 days of prednisolone was compared with placebo in the prevention of chronic nephropathy in a randomized trial [19]. However, the treatment did not prevent the development of chronic kidney disease. Thus, steroids have a limited role, if any, in HSP nephritis.

IgA Nephropathy

IgA nephropathy is seen in a small number of children [20]. It is often diagnosed with recurrent attacks of macroscopic hematuria and often microscopic hematuria between the attacks. The role of steroid treatment is very limited. A small group develops rapidly progressing GN, where this treatment might play a role.

Crescentic Nephritis

Rapidly progressive nephritis is a very uncommon diagnosis in children. On kidney biopsy samples, it is seen as a crescentic nephritis with features of another underlying GN of any kind. The treatment of rapidly progressive nephritis is often a combination of several immunosuppressive drugs including pulses of intravenous methylprednisolone and high doses of oral steroids [21].

Vasculitides

The most common vasculitis with renal involvement in childhood is HSP. Others, which occur infrequently in children, are antineutrophil cytoplasmic antibody (ANCA)-positive glomerulonephritis and polyarteritis nodosa.

ANCA-Positive Vasculitis

ANCA-positive vasculitis is a highly uncommon and very severe disease in children. With the help of the clinical picture and the occurrence of different ANCA patterns, it is grouped into microscopic polyangiitis and granulomatosis with polyangiitis (formerly Wegener's granulomatosis) [22–24]. These children are typically very unwell at presentation with major fatigue and weight loss and they are at high risk of rapid and often permanent loss of kidney function.

Children with an ANCA-associated vasculitis are initially treated in a similar way because they are extremely unwell and in urgent need of effective treatment. Initial pulses of methylprednisolone followed by high doses of oral prednisolone form a crucial part of this treatment [25].

Polyarteritis Nodosa

Polyarteritis nodosa is another quite uncommon vasculitic disease [26]. It normally presents with severe generalized symptoms and a marked vasculitic rash. The diagnosis is made from the clinical picture with the confirmation of vasculitis on a biopsy (often skin or kidney) and/or intrarenal vascular changes often with aneurysms [24].

The steroid treatment is very similar to that of any severe autoimmune disease with methylprednisolone and oral prednisolone. As always, the aim is to wean the steroids as soon as the clinical picture allows, but most children will need year-long treatment with a low dose. In many cases this can be achieved as alternate-day treatment that reduces the side effects.

Other Diagnoses

Children can be treated with steroids in a small number of other renal diagnoses, including tubulointerstitial nephritis (TIN). Children with acute pyelonephritis have also experimentally been treated with the aim of avoiding later renal scarring.

Tubulointerstitial Nephritis

TIN is a very uncommon condition during childhood. There are several causes for this including a reaction to drug treatment and an autoimmune condition [27]. Drug-induced TIN is often self-limiting if the drug is stopped. Patients with autoimmune TIN in many cases have symptoms also from other organ systems, typically uveitis (TINU). TINU is usually treated with steroids in a similar way as other autoimmune renal conditions [27].

Acute Pyelonephritis

Acute pyelonephritis is a bacterial infection in the renal parenchyma and is not normally treated with steroids but with the appropriate antibiotics [28]. A number of children, however, develop postinfectious scarring of the kidneys following one or several episodes of acute pyelonephritis [29]. Previous animal research and recent clinical studies have suggested that this renal scarring can be at least partly prevented by concomitant treatment with steroids during the acute phase of the renal infection [30]. However, many more well-designed studies are needed to make this an established treatment.

References

1. Eddy AA, Symons JM (2003) Nephrotic syndrome in childhood. Lancet 362:629–639
2. Arneil GC (1971) The nephrotic syndrome. Pediatr Clin North Am 18:547–559
3. Hodson EM, Knight JF, Willis NS, Craig JC (2000) Corticosteroid therapy in nephrotic syndrome: a meta-analysis of randomised controlled trials. Arch Dis Child 83:45–51
4. Teeninga N, Kist-van Holthe JE, van Rijswijk N et al (2013) Extending prednisolone treatment does not reduce relapses in childhood nephrotic syndrome. J Am Soc Nephrol 24:149–159
5. Hodson EM, Craig JC (2013) Corticosteroid therapy for steroid-sensitive nephrotic syndrome in children: dose or duration? J Am Soc Nephrol 24:7–9
6. Alternate-day versus intermittent prednisone in frequently relapsing nephrotic syndrome. A report of "Arbetsgemeinschaft fur Padiatrische Nephrologie" (1979). Lancet 1:401–403
7. Simmonds J, Grundy N, Trompeter R, Tullus K (2010) Long-term steroid treatment and growth: a study in steroid-dependent nephrotic syndrome. Arch Dis Child 95:146–149
8. Mori K, Honda M, Ikeda M (2004) Efficacy of methylprednisolone pulse therapy in steroid-resistant nephrotic syndrome. Pediatr Nephrol 19:1232–1236
9. Yorgin PD, Krasher J, Al-Uzri AY (2001) Pulse methylprednisolone treatment of idiopathic steroid-resistant nephrotic syndrome. Pediatr Nephrol 16:245–250
10. Fine RN (2007) Recurrence of nephrotic syndrome/focal segmental glomerulosclerosis following renal transplantation in children. Pediatr Nephrol 22:496–502
11. Rodriguez-Iturbe B, Musser JM (2008) The current state of poststreptococcal glomerulonephritis. J Am Soc Nephrol 19:1855–1864
12. Cameron JS (1994) Lupus nephritis in childhood and adolescence. Pediatr Nephrol 8:230–249

13. Tullus K (2012) New developments in the treatment of systemic lupus erythematosus. Pediatr Nephrol 27:727–732
14. Marks SD, Tullus K (2010) Modern therapeutic strategies for paediatric systemic lupus erythematosus and lupus nephritis. Acta Paediatr 99:967–974
15. Condon MB, Ashby D, Pepper RJ et al (2013) Prospective observational single-centre cohort study to evaluate the effectiveness of treating lupus nephritis with rituximab and mycophenolate mofetil but no oral steroids. Ann Rheum Dis 72:1280–1286
16. McCarthy HJ, Tizard EJ (2010) Clinical practice: diagnosis and management of Henoch-Schonlein purpura. Eur J Pediatr 169:643–650
17. Ruperto N, Ozen S, Pistorio A et al (2010) EULAR/PRINTO/PRES criteria for Henoch-Schonlein purpura, childhood polyarteritis nodosa, childhood Wegener granulomatosis and childhood Takayasu arteritis: Ankara 2008. Part I: Overall methodology and clinical characterisation. Ann Rheum Dis 69:790–797
18. Davin JC, Weening JJ (2003) Diagnosis of Henoch-Schonlein purpura: renal or skin biopsy? Pediatr Nephrol 18:1201–1203
19. Dudley J, Smith G, Llewelyn-Edwards A, Bayliss K, Pike K, Tizard J (2013) Randomised, double-blind, placebo-controlled trial to determine whether steroids reduce the incidence and severity of nephropathy in Henoch-Schonlein Purpura (HSP). Arch Dis Child 98:756–763
20. Mitsioni A (2001) IgA nephropathy in children. Nephrol Dial Transplant 16(Suppl 6):123–125
21. Little MA, Pusey CD (2004) Rapidly progressive glomerulonephritis: current and evolving treatment strategies. J Nephrol 17(Suppl 8):S10–S19
22. Brogan P, Eleftheriou D, Dillon M (2010) Small vessel vasculitis. Pediatr Nephrol 25:1025–1035
23. Kallenberg CG (2014) The diagnosis and classification of microscopic polyangiitis. J Autoimmun 48–49:90–93
24. Ozen S, Pistorio A, Iusan SM et al (2010) EULAR/PRINTO/PRES criteria for Henoch-Schonlein purpura, childhood polyarteritis nodosa, childhood Wegener granulomatosis and childhood Takayasu arteritis: Ankara 2008. Part II: Final classification criteria. Ann Rheum Dis 69:798–806
25. Eleftheriou D, Melo M, Marks SD et al (2009) Biologic therapy in primary systemic vasculitis of the young. Rheumatology (Oxford) 48:978–986
26. Eleftheriou D, Dillon MJ, Tullus K et al (2013) Systemic polyarteritis nodosa in the young: a single-center experience over thirty-two years. Arthritis Rheum 65:2476–2485
27. Ulinski T, Sellier-Leclerc AL, Tudorache E, Bensman A, Aoun B (2012) Acute tubulointerstitial nephritis. Pediatr Nephrol 27:1051–1057
28. Tullus K (2012) What do the latest guidelines tell us about UTIs in children under 2 years of age. Pediatr Nephrol 27:509–511
29. Toffolo A, Ammenti A, Montini G (2012) Long-term clinical consequences of urinary tract infections during childhood: a review. Acta Paediatr 101:1018–1031
30. Huang YY, Chen MJ, Chiu NT, Chou HH, Lin KY, Chiou YY (2011) Adjunctive oral methylprednisolone in pediatric acute pyelonephritis alleviates renal scarring. Pediatrics 128: e496–e504

Corticosteroids in Neonatology: Postnatal Corticosteroids in Preterm Infants with Bronchopulmonary Dysplasia

Silvia Perugi and Carlo Dani

Introduction

Adequate pulmonary function is crucial for preterm infants. In addition to being structurally immature, the preterm lung is susceptible to injury resulting from different prenatal conditions and postnatal insults. Lung injury may result in impaired postnatal lung development, contributing to chronic lung disease, and many preterm infants who survive go on to develop this pathology. This is probably caused by persistent inflammation in the lungs, and thus chronic lung disease is a major problem for infants in neonatal intensive care units and is associated with higher mortality rates and worse long-term outcomes in survivors.

Chronic lung disease after preterm birth, also known as bronchopulmonary dysplasia (BPD), a major morbidity of the very preterm infant, is remarkably resistant to therapeutic interventions, and negatively affects neurodevelopmental outcomes. There is a complex interaction between lung injury, lung inflammation, lung repair, and altered lung development. Also, there are interactions between fetal, perinatal, and postnatal factors modulating lung injury.

Neonatal Lung Injury

Preterm birth is greatly associated with respiratory distress syndrome (RDS), caused by structural and functional immaturity of the newborn lung. In addition to simple structural immaturity, the preterm lung is susceptible to injury resulting from different prenatal conditions such as intrauterine growth restriction or oligohydramnios, genetic disposition, transition at birth, and postnatal procedures and insults such as

S. Perugi • C. Dani (✉)
Division of Neonatology, Careggi University Hospital of Florence, Florence, Italy
e-mail: cdani@unifi.it

R. Cimaz (ed.), *Systemic Corticosteroids for Inflammatory Disorders in Pediatrics*, DOI 10.1007/978-3-319-16056-6_14

mechanical ventilation–induced trauma from volume and pressure changes, extension of tissue and oxygen toxicity, sepsis, hypoxia, and others. These early alterations may interfere with lung development and therefore exert lasting effects on pulmonary plasticity and integrity, finally resulting in structural and functional impairment. Although growing experimental evidence can elucidate the link between lung injury, lung inflammation, lung repair, and altered lung development, the interactions between injurious insults and inflammatory stimuli on different levels are complex and remain to be fully understood [1]. Furthermore, recent findings support the hypothesis that chronic lung injury originating in this early period of life or even antenatally may indeed have long-term adverse respiratory effects, and studies report an association between chorioamnionitis and both recurrent wheezing and physician-diagnosed asthma [2]. In addition, young adult survivors of moderate and severe BPD may be left with residual functional and characteristic structural pulmonary abnormalities, most notably emphysema. The premise is that extremely preterm infants may have immature adrenal gland function, predisposing them to a relative adrenal insufficiency and inadequate anti-inflammatory capability during the first several weeks of life.

Benefits of Corticosteroids in Lung Inflammation

Since persistent inflammation of the lungs is the most likely cause, corticosteroid drugs have been used to either prevent or treat chronic lung disease because of their strong anti-inflammatory effects particularly in babies who cannot be weaned from assisted ventilation. The beneficial effects were a shorter time on the ventilator and less chronic lung disease, but the adverse effects included high blood pressure, bleeding from the stomach or bowel, perforation of the bowel, an excess of glucose in the bloodstream, and an increased risk of cerebral palsy at follow-up. There were significant benefits for the following outcomes: lower rates of failure to extubate and decreased risks of chronic lung disease at both 28 days' and 36 weeks' postnatal age; death or chronic lung disease at 28 days' and 36 weeks' postmenstrual postnatal age; patent ductus arteriosus; and retinopathy of prematurity, including severe forms of this condition. There were no significant differences in the rates of neonatal or subsequent mortality, infection, severe intraventricular hemorrhage, periventricular leukomalacia, necrotizing enterocolitis, or pulmonary hemorrhage. Gastrointestinal bleeding and intestinal perforation were significant adverse effects, and the risks of hyperglycemia, hypertension, hypertrophic cardiomyopathy, and growth failure were also increased.

Neurodevelopmental Outcomes

Long-term follow-up studies [3] report an increased risk of abnormal neurological findings and cerebral palsy. However, the methodological quality of the studies determining long-term outcomes is limited in some cases; the surviving children were assessed predominantly before school age, and no study was sufficiently powered to detect important adverse long-term neurosensory outcomes. There is a compelling need for the long-term follow-up and reporting of late outcomes, especially neurological and developmental outcomes, among surviving infants who participated in all the randomized trials of early postnatal corticosteroid treatment. Dexamethasone was used in most studies, and only few used hydrocortisone. In subgroup analyses by type of corticosteroid, most of the beneficial and harmful effects were attributable to dexamethasone; hydrocortisone had little effect on any outcomes except for an increase in intestinal perforation and a borderline reduction in patent ductus arteriosus. Hydrocortisone appears to have less neurological impact than dexamethasone, even with adjustment for dose equivalency [4].

There are certain biological differences between these agents that may be of neurological relevance. Hydrocortisone differs from dexamethasone as it has both mineralocorticoid and glucocorticoid actions. In animal models, dexamethasone, which binds only to glucocorticoid receptors, induced neuronal degeneration within the hippocampus. In humans, alterations in hippocampal volume and synaptic plasticity and associative memory were reported with dexamethasone in preterm infants [5]. High-dose postnatal dexamethasone treatment for BPD was associated with decreased brain volumes on magnetic resonance imaging at 18 years of age, specifically total brain tissue, cortical white matter, thalamus, and basal ganglia nuclei. Surprisingly, some studies found no significant differences in the hippocampus or cerebellum, which are brain areas with very high concentrations of glucocorticoid receptors. Even in the absence of significant postnatal medical sequelae, preterm birth has a profound effect on neuroanatomical structures in childhood and adolescence [6–8]. Some authors have reported that individuals born extremely preterm have smaller brain volumes than term-born controls at 18 years of age, including the hippocampus and cerebellum as well as other brain regions; other authors have reported similar findings following preterm birth, including extremely preterm infants without "serious neurologic or medical conditions" at 7–10 years of age. They found that these children had smaller total brain volumes, white and gray matter volumes, and smaller basal ganglia and thalami than term-born controls [6–8]. These studies highlight the difficulty of distinguishing the effects of prematurity and its complications from the effects of a specific therapeutic intervention.

The differences observed in neurodevelopmental outcomes may result from the different effects of these agents on the hippocampus, an area of the brain critical for learning, memory, and spatial processing. The hippocampus contains a high density of both mineralocorticoid and glucocorticoid receptors. Hydrocortisone, which is identical to native cortisol, can bind to both classes of receptors. By contrast, dexamethasone binds only to glucocorticoid receptors, and in animal models this has been shown to result in degeneration and necrosis of hippocampal neurons.

It is also hypothesized that the longer biological half-life of dexamethasone relative to hydrocortisone influences potency and potential adverse effects, because it could have a much higher relative potency [9, 10].

Late steroid treatment (after 7 days of life) was associated with a reduction in neonatal mortality (at 28 days), but not mortality at discharge or latest reported age. Benefits of delayed steroid treatment included reductions in failure to extubate by 3, 7, or 28 days, chronic lung disease at both 28 days' and 36 weeks' postnatal age, need for late rescue treatment with dexamethasone, discharge on home oxygen, and death or chronic lung disease at both 28 days' and 36 weeks' postmenstrual postnatal age. There was a trend toward an increase in risk of infection and gastrointestinal bleeding, but not necrotizing enterocolitis. Short-term adverse effects included hyperglycemia, glycosuria, and hypertension. There was an increase in severe retinopathy of prematurity, but no significant increase in blindness. The trends toward an increase in cerebral palsy or abnormal neurological findings were partly offset by a trend in the opposite direction in death before late follow-up, but the combined rate of death or cerebral palsy was not significantly different between the steroid and control groups [11].

However, key messages continue to resonate following these studies and the policy statement of the American Academy of Pediatrics is that high doses of dexamethasone (>0.25 mg/kg/dose or >1.0 mg/kg total) should be avoided owing to their adverse neurological consequences because of reduced brain volume and increased disability; low-dose dexamethasone (0.15 mg/kg/dose commence or total 0.9 mg/kg) may help extubation but does not improve survival or BPD, and it reduces brain volumes but does not increase early disability. Moreover, low-dose (1–2 mg/kg/day) and high-dose hydrocortisone (3–6 mg/kg/day) after the first week of life do not seem to increase neurological risk, but have not been shown to improve rates of survival without BPD. Despite this concern over efficacy and safety, and despite the uncertainty, systemic corticosteroids remain a common treatment in very preterm infants: Close to 7 % of all preterm infants receive dexamethasone and 7 % receive hydrocortisone. Clinicians need guidance in balancing the risks against the benefits because both BPD and corticosteroids are associated with adverse long-term neurologic outcomes: Lung disease itself, without any glucocorticoid therapy, results in anomalies in brain white matter development and BPD is also linked to adverse neurodevelopmental outcomes. In addition, BPD is highly variable; even within this diagnosis, it is likely that sicker babies are more often treated with dexamethasone, and those babies are also more likely to have worse outcomes.

Thus, a proper approach to the problem is to consider if the risks and benefits of corticosteroid treatment might vary with the underlying risk of developing BPD. To this end, data available from randomized controlled trials showed that the effect of systemic corticosteroids on the combined outcome of death or cerebral palsy was negatively related to the rate of BPD in the control group. Therefore, if the rate of BPD in the control group was low, the steroid treatment was harmful, while if the rate of BPD in the control group was high, there was benefit and an increased incidence of survival free of cerebral palsy. Thus, clinicians who need guidance on whether to start systemic steroid therapy in ventilator-dependent infants could use their own local data for the risk of BPD to identify the highest-risk infants who might have an actual benefit from treatment.

No randomized controlled trials of other systemic glucocorticoids, such as prednisone or methylprednisolone, to treat or prevent BPD have been published. Moreover, no additional evidence has been published to support the efficacy of inhaled glucocorticoids in preventing or decreasing the severity of BPD [11].

Conclusions

The benefits of *early* postnatal corticosteroid treatment (first 7 days of life), particularly dexamethasone, may not outweigh the adverse effects of this treatment. Although early corticosteroid treatment facilitates extubation and reduces the risk of BPD and patent ductus arteriosus, it causes short-term adverse effects including gastrointestinal bleeding, intestinal perforation, hyperglycemia, hypertension, hypertrophic cardiomyopathy, and growth failure. Long-term follow-up studies report an increased risk of abnormal neurological findings and cerebral palsy, but long-term outcome data are limited; the surviving children were assessed predominantly before school age, and no study was sufficiently powered to detect important adverse long-term neurosensory outcomes. There is a compelling need for the long-term follow-up and reporting of late outcomes, especially neurological and developmental outcomes, among surviving infants who participated in all the randomized trials of early postnatal corticosteroid treatment. The beneficial or the harmful effects of hydrocortisone are few, and it cannot be recommended for the prevention of chronic lung disease. Use of early corticosteroids, especially dexamethasone, to treat or prevent chronic lung disease should be curtailed until more research has been performed [12].

Postnatal *late* corticosteroid treatment for chronic lung disease initiated after 7 days of age may reduce neonatal mortality without significantly increasing the risk of adverse long-term neurodevelopmental outcomes, but the methodological quality of the studies determining the long-term outcome is limited and the surviving children were been assessed before school age, when some important neurological outcomes cannot be determined with certainty. Moreover, no study was sufficiently powered to detect increased rates of important adverse long-term neurosensory outcomes. On the other hand, postnatal late corticosteroid treatment at high doses is associated with short-term side effects such as bleeding from the stomach or bowel, higher blood pressure, and glucose intolerance.

Given the evidence of both benefits and harms of systemic postnatal steroidal treatment, it seems important to reserve the use of late corticosteroids for those infants who cannot be weaned from mechanical ventilation and to minimize the dose and duration of treatment. Considering the existing data, we believe that early postnatal corticosteroids are harmful and should not be further tested. Conversely, we should consider trials for infants who cannot be extubated by 14–21 days, who are at significant risk of developing BPD. Such trials must be large enough to measure the impact of steroids on both pulmonary outcomes and important long-term developmental outcomes. In fact, the American Academy of Pediatrics in 2010 stated that very low-birth-weight infants who remain on mechanical ventilation after 1–2 weeks of age are at very high risk of developing BPD. When considering corticosteroid therapy for these infants, clinicians might conclude that the risks of a short course of glucocorticoids to mitigate BPD are justified. This individualized decision should be made in conjunction with the infant's parents [13].

References

1. Doyle LW, Ehrenkranz RA, Halliday HL (2014) Early (<8 days) postnatal corticosteroids for preventing chronic lung disease in preterm infants. Cochrane Database Syst Rev 5:CD001146
2. Hütten MC, Kramer BW (2014) Patterns and etiology of acute and chronic lung injury: insights from experimental evidence. Chin J Contemp Pediatr 16(5):448–459
3. Benders M (2013) Postnatal steroids in the preterm infant—the good, the ugly, and the unknown. J Pediatr 162:667–669
4. Stark AR, Carlo WA, Vohr BR, Papile LA, Saha S, Bauer CR et al (2014) Death or neurodevelopmental impairment at 18 to 22 months in a randomized trial of early dexamethasone to prevent death or chronic lung disease in extremely low birth weight infants. J Pediatr 164(1):34–39
5. DeMauro SB, Dysart K, Kirpalani H (2014) Stopping the swinging pendulum of postnatal corticosteroid use. J Pediatr 164:9–10
6. Doyle LW, Ehrenkranz RA, Halliday HL (2014) Late (>7 days) postnatal corticosteroids for chronic lung disease in preterm infants. Cochrane Database Syst Rev 5:CD001145
7. Doyle Lex W, Sinclair JC et al (2014) An update on the impact of postnatal systemic corticosteroids on mortality and cerebral palsy in preterm infants: effect modification by risk of bronchopulmonary dysplasia. J Pediatr 165(6):1258–1260
8. Greenberg SB (2014) Dexamethasone and the brain at age 18 years: randomize the first baby and follow-up. J Pediatr 164(4):687–689
9. Cheong JL, Burnett AC, Lee KJ, Roberts G, Thompson DK, Wood SJ, Victorian Infant Collaborative Study Group et al (2014) Association between postnatal dexamethasone for treatment of bronchopulmonary dysplasia and brain volumes at adolescence in infants born very preterm. J Pediatr 164(4):737–743
10. Cheong JL, Anderson PJ, Roberts G, Burnett AC, Lee KJ, Thompson DK et al (2013) Contribution of brain size to IQ and educational underperformance in extremely preterm adolescents. PLoS One 8(10):e77475
11. Gupta S, Prasanth K, Yeh FT (2012) Postnatal corticosteroids for prevention and treatment of chronic lung disease in the preterm newborn. Int J Pediatr 2012:315642
12. Patra K, Greene MM, Silvestri JM (2014) Neurodevelopmental impact of hydrocortisone exposure in extremely low birth weight infants: outcomes at 1 and 2 years. J Perinatol 35(1):77–81
13. American Academy of Pediatrics (2010) Postnatal corticosteroids to prevent or treat bronchopulmonary dysplasia. Pediatrics 126(4):800–808

MIX
Papier aus verantwortungsvollen Quellen
Paper from responsible sources
FSC® C105338

If you have any concerns about our products,
you can contact us on
ProductSafety@springernature.com

In case Publisher is established outside the EU,
the EU authorized representative is:
Springer Nature Customer Service Center GmbH
Europaplatz 3, 69115 Heidelberg, Germany

Printed by Libri Plureos GmbH
in Hamburg, Germany